P9-BYG-733

ACROMEGALY AND ITS MANAGEMENT

Acromegaly and Its Management

Alan G. Harris, M.D.
Department of Medicine
Dijkzigt University Hospital
Erasmus University
Rotterdam, The Netherlands

SCIENTIFIC EDITOR

Adrian F. Daly, B.Sc.
Royal College of Surgeons in Ireland
Dublin, Ireland

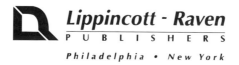

Lippincott - Raven
PUBLISHERS

Philadelphia • New York

Lippincott-Raven Publishers, **227 E**ast Washington Square,
Philadelphia, Pennsylvania **19106**

© 1996 Lippincott-Raven Publishers. All rights reserved. This book is protected by
copyright. No part of it may be reproduced, stored in a retrieval system, or transmitted,
in any form or by any means, electronic, mechanical, photocopying, or recording, or
otherwise, without the prior written permission of the publisher.

Made in the United States of America

ISBN 0-397-51814-5

The material contained in this volume was submitted as previously unpublished material, except in the instances in which credit has been given to the source from which
some of the illustrative material was derived. Illustrations provided courtesy of Sandoz
Pharma Ltd.

Great care has been taken to maintain the accuracy of the information contained in the
volume. However, neither Lippincott-Raven Publishers nor the author nor the editor can
be held responsible for errors or for any consequences arising from the use of the information contained herein.

Materials appearing in this book prepared by individuals as part of their official duties
as U.S. Government employees are not covered by the above-mentioned copyright.

9 8 7 6 5 4 3 2 1

Cover: [^{111}In]DTPA octreotide scintigraphy of a GH secreting pituitary adenoma courtesy of Prof. E. P. Krenning, Erasmus University Rotterdam, The Netherlands.

Contents

Foreword

The pathologic effects of excess growth hormone secretion are as diverse as they are profound. The impact of acromegaly on the patient is enormous, decreasing both life expectancy and quality of life. Endocrine, metabolic, cardiovascular, and musculoskeletal changes associated with acromegaly cause significant perturbation of normal physiologic processes, and the combined effects of physical deformity and chronic illness play havoc with patients' psychological health. Thankfully, as we approach the new millennium, advances in basic science and therapy have provided clinicians with tools that allow early diagnosis and strict control of acromegaly. Other ongoing work continues to highlight the biology of insidious changes associated with acromegaly. Data from epidemiologic and outcome studies show us that our past criteria for "cure" in acromegaly may need to be further refined. Until treatment is able to transform the pathologic activity of a growth hormone–secreting adenoma to the patterns seen in normal patients, the transition from disease "control" to "cure" will not have been made.

In this book on acromegaly, I hope to provide the reader with a volume that is both comprehensive and readable. For the specialist, the book provides a contemporary distillation of our knowledge to date concerning all aspects of acromegaly. For general clinicians, residents, and medical students, it is intended that this work will encapsulate the essentials of acromegaly and its management in a readily understood manner. I hope that this volume will help to increase general awareness of acromegaly throughout the medical community so that we can hasten diagnosis and improve the treatment of patients suffering from acromegaly in the future.

Acromegaly proves the old adage that physicians should have "a high index of clinical suspicion," because if acromegaly is not considered as a diagnosis, the patient may be condemned to many years of confusion and suffering. All should realize that once acromegaly is suspected, then confirming it or discarding it as a diagnosis is eminently easy and is almost entirely painless.

My thanks go to Prof. Steven Lamberts, who has doubly honored me by reviewing the content of this book and by kindly agreeing to write the preface. I also thank Drs. A. Beckers (Liege, Belgium), M. Bergstrom (Uppsala, Sweden), K. Ho (Sydney, Australia), P. O. Lundberg (Uppsala, Sweden), E. P. Krenning (Rotterdam, The Netherlands), C. Muhr (Uppsala, Sweden), S. Reichlin (Boston, U.S.A.), J. C. Reubi (Berne, Switzerland), A. Stadnik (Brussels, Belgium), A. Stevenaert (Liege, Belgium), J. P. Tauber (Toulouse, France), and my other colleagues who provided me with photographs of their patients and illustrations from their collections. I gratefully acknowledge the efforts of Anthony Fazio and Kathleen Felix at Lippincott–Raven Publishers. Finally, I am grateful to my colleague Adrian Daly, who collaborated closely with me to define and encapsulate the essential scientific and clinical elements in the chapters that follow.

Preface

Acromegaly is a disease that has intrigued and fascinated mankind throughout the ages. Although the overt manifestations of soft tissue swelling and bony overgrowth are distressing, patients also suffer from significant long-term morbidity and mortality due to respiratory and cardiovascular disease, as well as cancer. In recent times, increasing emphasis has been placed on the early recognition of acromegaly, to prevent the development of the full-blown clinical picture. It has also become evident that whatever form of therapy is chosen for the individual patient, the primary goal should be the rapid and complete normalization of growth hormone secretion.

Dr. Harris has described thoroughly the clinical presentation and management of acromegaly, aided by excellent photographs and illustrations. The clinical work-up of the newly diagnosed patient, the different treatment options with their respective advantages and disadvantages, and the essentials of long-term follow-up care are well summarized. Acromegaly is a model of how recent developments in neuroscience, molecular biology, and pharmacotherapy have combined to advance the diagnosis and treatment of a disease. Dr. Harris has made a long-standing contribution to the development of medical therapy for patients with acromegaly, which has been translated admirably in this balanced and informative textbook.

Steven W. J. Lamberts M.D., Ph.D.
Professor of Medicine
Department of Medicine
University Hospital Dijkzigt
Erasmus University
Rotterdam, The Netherlands

Introduction

Acromegaly is a rare disease characterized by excessive skeletal growth and soft tissue enlargement. The word "acromegaly" is derived from the Greek words "akron," meaning extremity, and "megas," meaning great. Acromegaly and gigantism represent a disease process that is differentiated only by the age of onset. Patients who develop growth hormone (GH)–secreting pituitary tumors during childhood experience excessive growth of long bones because the epiphyses have not yet fused, a clinical syndrome known as gigantism. After puberty (and epiphyseal fusion), these patients can progress to exhibit all of the typical signs and symptoms of acromegaly if they remain untreated. In acromegaly proper, the disease often has an insidious onset and becomes overtly symptomatic when patients reach the third or fourth decade. In more than 95% of cases, acromegaly is caused by excessive secretion of GH by an adenoma of the anterior pituitary gland, with the remainder caused by hypothalamic or ectopic growth hormone-releasing hormone (GHRH)–secreting tumors.

The public in general and the medical profession in particular have long had a fascination with rare disorders. No group of diseases has attracted more attention during our history than the disorders of growth. Giants and dwarfs populate mythology and ancient history in almost every culture. Probably the most famous example is Goliath of the Bible, who was reported to be over 9 feet tall ("six cubits and a span").

During the 18th and 19th centuries, many people with pituitary gigantism suffered the ignominy of appearing as circus and sideshow attractions, sadly being viewed as freaks of nature rather than as patients suffering from an illness. Indeed, the medical profession was occasionally guilty of concentrating more on the novelty factor of excessive stature and less on the patient's needs. The best illustration of this is the famous story of Charles Byrne, whose skeleton now resides in the museum of the Royal College of Surgeons in London. Byrne, an Irishman who died in the late 18th century, was once billed as the "world's tallest man" and attracted the interest not only of the public at large but also of the surgeons and anatomists of London. In an attempt to avoid becoming a research specimen after his death, Byrne paid for disposal of his body in a weighted coffin in the Irish Sea. After his eventual death, however, the accomplices were halted almost in the final act of disposal and were persuaded (financially and alcoholically, of course) to hand Byrne's body over for dissection and study. It was later reported that Byrne's skull had an enlarged pituitary fossa, indicating that his excessive stature was probably due to a GH-secreting pituitary macroadenoma (1).

Thankfully, greater enlightenment found its way into medicine at the end of the 19th century, as interest in clinical research developed. In 1886, a French physician, Pierre Marie, described a noncongenital syndrome of increased growth of the face, hands, and feet in two patients, and termed this condition acromegaly (2). In the following year, Minkowski (3) suggested a causal relationship between pituitary pathology and acromegaly, but this view was not generally elucidated until the studies of Benda and Cushing during the first decade of the 20th century (4,5). Working with Davidoff, Harvey Cushing reported that in acromegaly the pituitary was usually enlarged by an "adenomatous" or "hyperplastic" process consisting of hormone-producing cells responsible for acromegaly (6). Effective treatment for acromegaly was instituted by Cushing with partial pituitary resection, at first via the frontal sinuses and later via the transsphenoidal route that is used to this day. Postoperative analysis of resected tumor material defined the link between tumor removal and remission of acromegalic signs and symptoms (7).

Our understanding of the etiology and natural history of acromegaly has advanced greatly since these early studies. New treatments and refinements of established therapies have been introduced, and patients now have the options of effective surgical, medical, and radiologic treatments. This book deals comprehensively with the pathogenesis and treatment of acromegaly. All treatment options for acromegaly (e.g., surgery, radiotherapy, pharmacotherapy) are assessed, with special emphasis on new developments in the field, such as somatostatin analogues, with which the general physician may not be familiar. Separate sections deal with the anatomy, physiology, and histology of the hypothalamus and the pituitary gland. Later chapters describe the epidemiology and pathogenesis of acromegaly, the diagnosis of the disease, and the pathologic changes that occur with chronically elevated levels of GH. Finally, all treatments for acromegaly, including surgery, radiotherapy, and medical treatment (somatostatin analogues and dopamine agonists) are described in detail. The impact of these treatments on hormone secretion, organic pathology, and on physical signs and symptoms of acromegaly are assessed. This book makes liberal use of illustrations and graphics to aid the reader and to underscore important points. A great deal of research on acromegaly has been published over the past few years, and this book attempts to provide a concise and up-to-date overview of current opinions concerning acromegaly, while maintaining readability and emphasizing the essentials of this disease.

REFERENCES

1. Keith A. An inquiry into the nature of the skeletal changes in acromegaly. *Lancet* 1911;1:993.
2. Marie P. Sur deux cas d'acromégalie: hypertrophie singuliére non congénitale des extrémitiés supérieures, inférieures et céphalique. *Rev Med* 1886;6:297–333.
3. Minkowski O. Über einen Fall von Akromegalie. *Berl Klin Wochensch* 1887;21:371–4.
4. Benda C. Beitrage zur normalen und pathologischen Histologie der menschlichen Hypophysis Cerebri. *Klin Wochensch* 1900;36:1205.
5. Cushing H. Partial hypophysectomy for acromegaly; with remarks on the function of the hypophysis. *Ann Surg* 1909;50:1002–17.
6. Cushing H, Davidoff LM. The pathological findings in four autopsied cases of acromegaly with a discussion of their significance. Monogr 22, Rockefeller Inst. Med. Research. New York: Waverly, 1927.
7. Bailey P, Davidoff LM. Concerning the microscopic structure of the hypophysis cerebri in acromegaly (based on a study of tissues removed at operation from 35 patients). *Am J Pathol* 1925;1:185–201.

ACROMEGALY AND ITS MANAGEMENT

CHAPTER 1

The Hypothalamic–Pituitary Axis

Although acromegaly is overwhelmingly a disease of the anterior pituitary, an adequate understanding of normal pituitary function also requires a discussion of the role of the hypothalamus. In phylogenetic terms, the hypothalamus is an old structure that plays a key role in the regulation of pituitary function. These two centers are so closely linked in the regulation of hormonal function that they are commonly referred to as the hypothalamic–pituitary axis. A correct understanding of the governing role of the hypothalamus over anterior pituitary function has come only in comparatively recent times with the work of Guillemin's (1,2) and Schally's (3,4) groups, for which they were awarded the Nobel Prize for Medicine or Physiology in 1977.

THE HYPOTHALAMUS

Gross Anatomy

The hypothalamus is a small structure, weighing 2.5–5.0 g and measuring approximately 1.5 cm in diameter. It is derived from a swelling on the developing diencephalon at 5–6 weeks of gestation, with the full structure becoming delineated by 8 weeks, by which time it has joined with the embryonic pituitary. Nerve cell axons grow from the hypothalamus through the pituitary stalk to help form the posterior pituitary (neurohypophysis) by the end of the second trimester. As shown in Fig. 1, the hypothalamus is a part of the diencephalon and is bounded superiorly and inferiorly by the thalamus and the pituitary, respectively. Its anterosuperior border is the anterior commissure, and it is bounded anteroinferiorly by the region comprising the optic chiasm and the lamina terminalis. The posterior border of the hypothalamus consists of the posterior parts of the mamillary bodies and the tegmentum of the midbrain. The lateral borders are complex and have been described variously as being formed by the optic tracts, internal capsule, the globus pallidus, the subthalamic nucleus, the cerebral peduncle, and the ansa lenticularis. Behind the hypothalamus runs the III ventricle, communicating with the lateral ventricle above and the IV ventricle below via the foramen of Munroe and the aqueduct of Silvius, respectively.

Blood Supply and Innervation

The hypothalamus receives its arterial supply from the internal carotid artery (via the circle of Willis) and the hypophyseal arteries. These vessels form an internal and an external plexus of capillaries, which feed into a portal network that drains into a network of vessels surrounding the anterior pituitary. The hypothalamus is innervated by many regions of the brain, including the limbic system, the brainstem, the thalamus, and the visual cortex. Efferent fibers connect various hypothalamic nuclei with the thalamus, midbrain, brainstem, spinal cord, and posterior pituitary gland.

Hypothalamic nerve endings within the median eminence secrete releasing or inhibitory factors into the portal vasculature, where they pass to the anterior pituitary to mediate their effects. The precise distribution of the vasculature and nerves within the hypothalamus is extremely complex and is beyond the scope of this publication. For a more detailed description, a review has been published by Scheithauer (5).

THE PITUITARY GLAND

Gross Anatomy

The pituitary gland, or hypophysis, weighs between 0.5 and 1.0 g and has dimensions of approximately $13 \times 9 \times 6$ mm. It consists of two parts, the larger anterior gland (ca. 80%) and the smaller posterior gland (ca. 20%). The pituitary lies within the sella turcica, a depression in the sphenoid bone of the skull that is lined with dura. The dura itself is reflected backwards to cover the superior border of the anterior pituitary, and is called the diaphragma sellae.

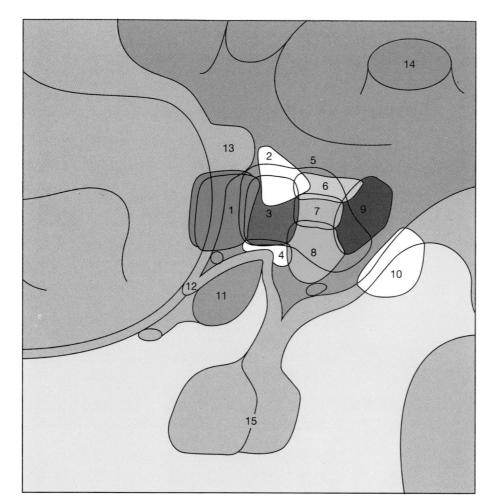

FIG. 1. Sagittal section of hypothalamic nuclei. 1, Preoptic nucleus; 2, paraventricular nucleus; 3, anterior hypothalamic area; 4, supraoptic nucleus; 5, lateral hypothalamic area; 6, dorsal hypothalamic area; 7, dorsomedial nucleus; 8, ventromedial nucleus; 9, posterior hypothalamic area; 10, mamillary body; 11, optic chiasm; 12, lamina terminalis; 13, anterior commissure; 14, interthalamic adhesion; 15, pituitary gland.

An aperture in the diaphragma sellae allows passage of the pituitary stalk that connects the pituitary with the hypothalamus above (Figs. 2–4). At about 6 weeks of fetal life, the pituitary is derived from two separate structures, an upgrowth from the endodermal Rathke's pouch, which is part of the stomodeum (forming the anterior pituitary or adenohypophysis), and a downgrowth of neuroectodermal tissue from the hypothalamus (forming the posterior pituitary).

Cryosection Studies

The development of rapid frozen sectioning (cryosectioning) techniques has been one of the most important advances in pathology in recent times. Muhr (6) has applied modified cryosectioning and cryomicrotomy to analysis of normal variations in pituitary anatomy (Fig. 5). This series of 40 autopsy specimens provides detailed information about variations in the structure and relations of the normal pituitary gland preserved in an intact state. Interestingly, in 15 cases with radiologic evidence of minor changes in cor-

tical bone or a sloping sellar floor, no expansive lesion of the pituitary gland was found. This knowledge is important for detailed evaluation of roentgenograms, computerized tomograms (CT) and magnetic resonance imaging (MRI), as well as for accurate focusing of new stereotactic radiosurgical procedures.

Blood Supply and Innervation

As outlined above, arterial blood containing releasing and inhibitory factors flows from the portal vessels of the hypothalamus to a plexus surrounding the anterior pituitary (Fig. 6). From this plexus, capillary sinusoids enter the body of the anterior pituitary. Venous drainage occurs mainly via the cavernous and petrosal sinuses, along with venous blood from the posterior portion of the gland. The anterior pituitary is sparsely innervated by the fine sympathetic nerves of the carotid plexus, which serve a vasomotor function. The posterior lobe receives rich innervation from the supraopticohypophyseal and tuberohypophyseal tracts, both of which originate from nuclei of the hypothalamus

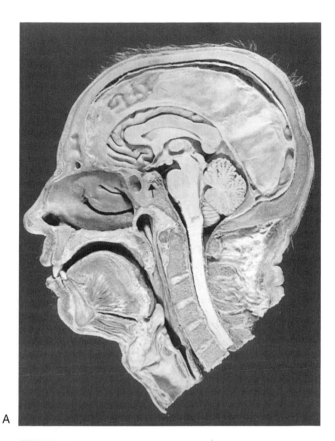

A

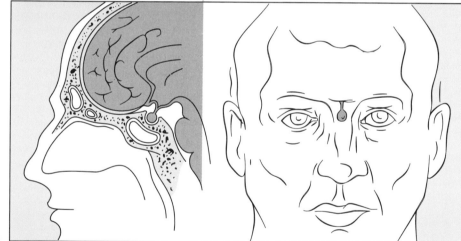

B

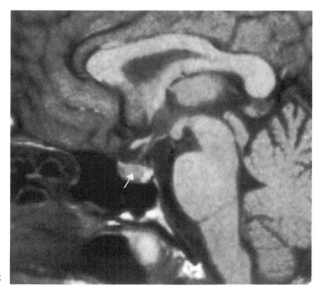

C

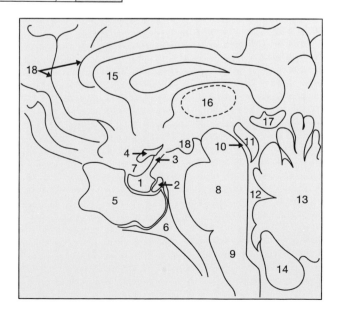

FIG. 2. **A:** Sagittal section of the head showing the pituitary gland *(arrow)*. **B:** Schematic representation of the pituitary gland. **C:** Midsagittal magnetic resonance imaging (MRI) section of the brain showing the pituitary. 1, Adenohypophysis; 2, neurohypophysis; 3, pituitary stalk; 4, optic chiasm; 5, sphenoid sinus; 6, clinus; 7, suprasellar cistern; 8, pons; 9, medulla oblongata; 10, aqueduct; 11, tectum mesencephali; 12, 4th ventricle; 13, cerebellum; 14, tonsil; 15, corpus callosum; 16, thalamus; 17, pineal gland; 18, cortical grooves. (MRI courtesy of A. Stadnik.)

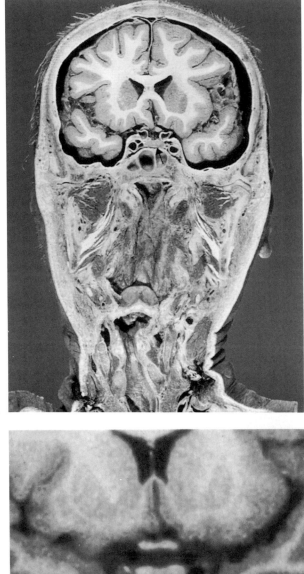

A

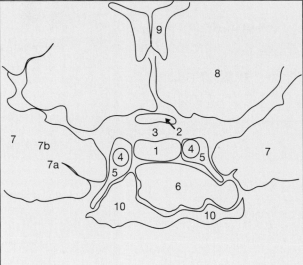

B

FIG. 3. **A:** Frontal section of the head showing the pituitary gland *(arrow)*. **B:** Coronal MRI section of the brain showing the pituitary. The CSF (cerebrospinal fluid) is dark, the white matter is bright and the grey matter has an intermediate signal. The adenohypophysis is isointense with the chiasm. 1, (Adeno)hypophysis; 2, chiasm; 3, suprasellar cistern; 4, carotid artery; 5, cavernous sinus; 6, sphenoid sinus; 7, temporal lobe; 7a, grey matter; 7b, white matter; 8, frontal lobe; 9, frontal horn; 10, bone (clinus). (Courtesy of A. Stadnik.)

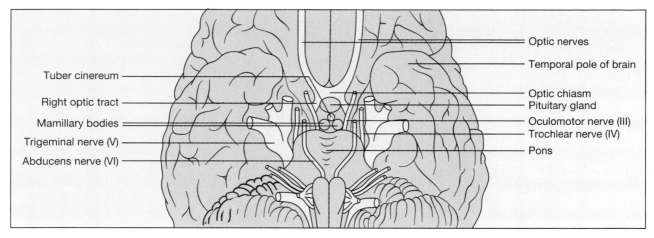

Tuber cinereum

Right optic tract

Mamillary bodies

Trigeminal nerve (V)

Abducens nerve (VI)

Optic nerves

Temporal pole of brain

Optic chiasm
Pituitary gland

Oculomotor nerve (III)

Trochlear nerve (IV)

Pons

FIG. 4. Interior view of the pituitary.

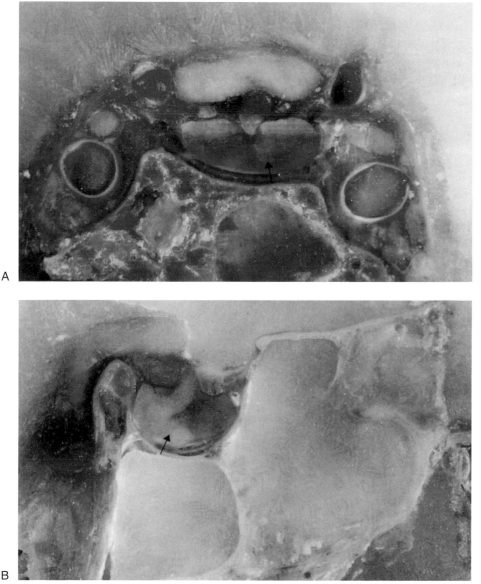

A

B

FIG. 5. Frontal **(A)** and sagittal **(B)** cryosection through the sellar region. (Courtesy of C. Muhr, University of Uppsala, Sweden.)

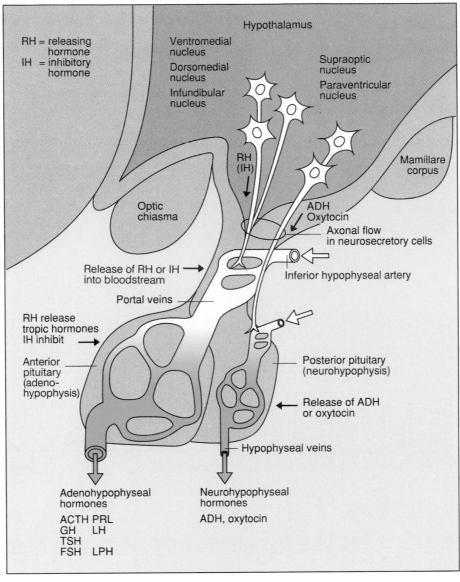

FIG. 6. Blood supply and innervation of the pituitary.

and are responsible for secretion of the hormones vasopressin and oxytocin.

Histology

Light microscopy combined with traditional staining methods allow a distinction to be made only between acidic (acidophilic), basic (basophilic), and nonstaining (chromophobic) anterior pituitary cells. This technique is nonspecific and, in the case of chromophobic cells, groups together cells that have divergent secretory roles. More precise immunohistochemical techniques have revealed the presence of five main cell populations in the normal anterior pituitary gland (Fig. 7):

Somatotrophs (±50% of total) produce GH (somatotropin) and are located in the lateral borders of the pituitary (Figs. 8 and 9).
Lactotrophs (15–20% of total) secrete prolactin (PRL) and are believed to arise, with somatotrophs, from a com-

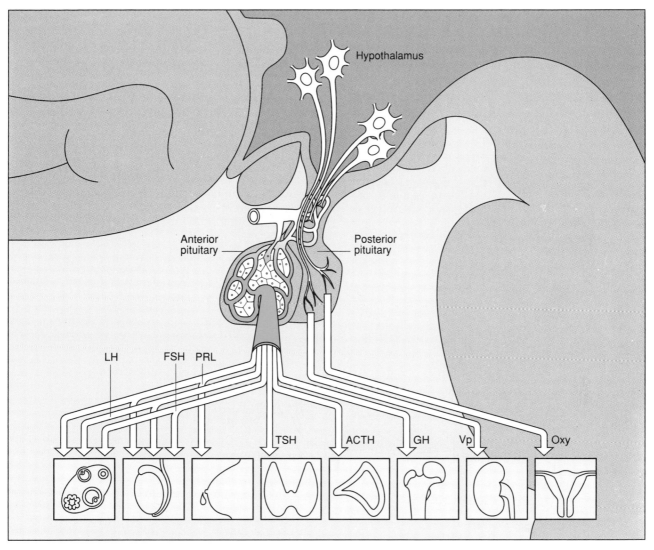

FIG. 7. Pituitary function: peripheral effects of pituitary hormones. LH, luteinizing hormone; FSH, folli-cle-stimulating hormone; PRL, prolactin; TSH, thyroid-stimulating hormone; ACTH, adrenocortico-tropic hormone; GH, growth hormone; Vp, vasopressin; Oxy, oxytocin.

mon progenitor cell. Some cells produce both GH and PRL and are termed somatomammotrophs. They are also located in the lateral areas of the gland.

Corticotrophs (10–20% of total) are found at a number of sites within the pituitary (mainly in the center) and are responsible for the production of a adrenocorticotrophic hormone (ACTH), melanocyte-stimulating hormone (MSH), β-lipoprotein hormone (β-LPH), and β-endor-phin from a common precursor molecule, pro-opiome-lanocortin (POMC).

Thyrotrophs (5–10% of total) secrete thyroid-stimulating hormone (TSH) and are found both on the surface of the gland and scattered within the core.

Gonadotrophs (5–10%) can produce both follicle-stimulat-ing hormone (FSH) and luteinizing hormone (LH), and are found in close relation to prolactin-secreting cells.

The histologic classification of the pituitary is by no means complete because certain cell types remain unidentified, and these may be responsible for the secretion of other pituitary factors of which we are at present unaware.

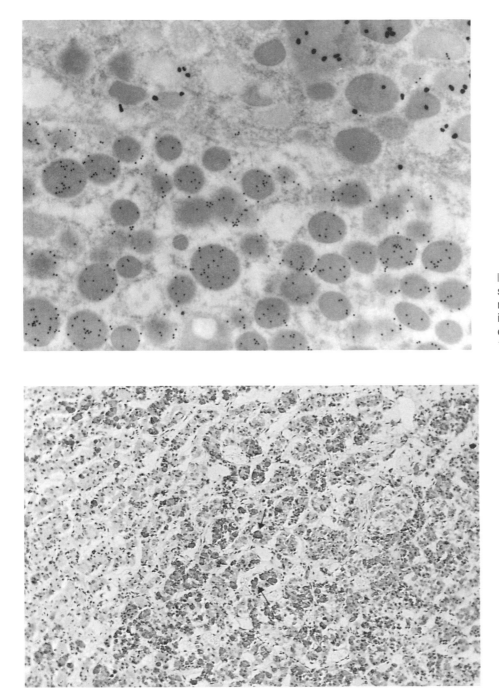

FIG. 8. Double gold immunostaining showing GH (15 n*M*) and PRL (40 n*M*) producing cells in a normal pituitary (electron microscope × 25,000; courtesy of A. Beckers, *Acta Endocr* 1988;118:503–12, with permission).

FIG. 9. Growth hormone as revealed by optical immunocytochemistry (PAP method) in the normal pituitary. (Courtesy of A. Beckers, loc. cit.)

REFERENCES

1. Guillemin R, Brazeau P, Bohlen P, et al. Growth hormone-releasing factor from a human pancreatic tumor that caused acromegaly. *Science* 1982;218:585.
2. Brazeau P, Vale W, Burgus R, et al. Hypothalamic polypeptide that inhibits the secretion of immunoreactive pituitary growth hormone. *Science* 1973;179:77–9.
3. Baba Y, Matsuo H, Schally AV. Structure of the porcine LH- and FSH-releasing hormone II. Confirmation of the proposed structure by conventional sequential analysis. *Biochem Biophys Res Commun* 1971; 44:459–67.
4. Schally AV, Arimura A, Baba Y, et al. Isolation and properties of the FSH and LH releasing hormone. *Biochem Biophys Res Commun* 1971; 43:393–9.
5. Scheithauer BW. The hypothalamus and neurohypophysis. In: Kovacs K, Asa SL, eds. *Functional endocrine pathology*. Vol. 1. Boston: Blackwell Scientific Publications, 1991:170–244.
6. Muhr C. The sella turcica and the pituitary gland: normal variations and diagnostic aspects of pituitary adenomas. Doctoral Thesis, University of Uppsala, 1981.

CHAPTER 2

Physiology of Growth Hormone

STRUCTURE, SYNTHESIS, AND SECRETION

Human growth hormone (GH, somatotropin) is a single-chain polypeptide consisting of 191 amino acids (MW 22,000) and containing two intramolecular disulfide bonds. It is synthesized as a intracellular prohormone before being secreted in the biologically active form. Two splice variants of GH have been characterized, a 22-kDa and a 20-kDa form, which constitute approximately 90% and 10% of GH in the pituitary gland, respectively. Both have identical biologic actions. Although the 191–amino-acid form is the predominant type of GH found in the body, two larger, possibly polymeric forms, termed "big" and "big–big" GH, have been reported (1). The role of these larger forms of GH is unclear at this time.

GH is manufactured and secreted by the somatotrophic and somatomammotrophic cells of the lateral anterior pituitary. The genes for GH expression are located on chromosome 17 (2). At any given time, the anterior pituitary gland contains up to 5–10 mg of GH (3), stored in intracellular granules or still attached to ribosomes. Another source of GH is GH-V, which is secreted by the placenta in pregnancy and is coded for by the GH-V gene (4). GH-V takes over from pituitary GH during late pregnancy and is the main determinant of circulating insulin-like growth factor-I (IGF-I) (see below) during pregnancy in both healthy and acromegalic women (5,6).

GH is secreted in a pulsatile manner every 2–4 h, with plasma levels rising from a baseline concentration of <1 μg/L to peaks as high as 25–50 μg/L. Most GH is secreted at night, in synchrony with deep sleep (7) (stage III/IV) (Fig. 10), but it is also secreted in response to exercise and other forms of physical stress (8). Control of GH secretion is complex (see below), but is mainly under the influence of the hypothalamic hormones growth hormone-releasing hormone (GHRH) and somatostatin, which stimu-

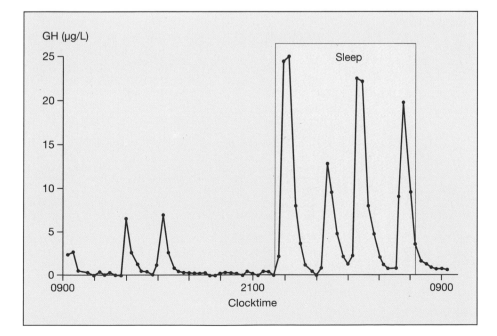

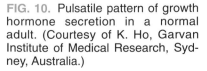

FIG. 10. Pulsatile pattern of growth hormone secretion in a normal adult. (Courtesy of K. Ho, Garvan Institute of Medical Research, Sydney, Australia.)

late and inhibit GH release, respectively. Women secrete approximately 500 μg/m^2 of GH per day, whereas men have a lower rate of secretion, at around 350 μg/m^2/day. Age-related variations in GH secretory rates also occur (9), with the rate being highest in adolescents and lowest in individuals over 50–60 years of age (10).

GH has a plasma half-life of 20–25 min and is cleared at a rate of 100–150 ml/m^2 body surface area. Elimination of GH is independent of both age and sex and occurs almost exclusively via the liver, with a small amount excreted in the urine. Plasma total free GH levels, obesity, and renal function have recently been shown to be determinants of GH elimination in humans, whereas age is a factor only at supraphysiologic GH concentrations, which is an important fact to note in acromegalic patients (11).

CONTROL OF NORMAL GROWTH HORMONE SECRETION

Episodic GH secretion is regulated primarily by the dynamic interaction of the two hypothalamic hormones, GHRH and somatostatin. However, there are many other factors that modulate GH secretion directly at the level of the hypothalamus, the pituitary gland, or both. These factors can be loosely categorized as hormonal, metabolic, and neurologic.

Hypothalamic Regulation of GH Secretion

GH secretion is regulated by a number of hormones, including GHRH, somatostatin, glucocorticoids, and thyroid hormones (T$_3$ and T$_4$). After remaining elusive for many years, GHRH was characterized in the early 1980s from pancreatic endocrine tumor tissue. It is a short molecule, composed of 44 amino acids, and is cleaved from a large precursor (12). The GHRH-secreting neurons are found in the infundibular nucleus and the median eminence (13). Somatostatin is a short molecule, consisting of 14

amino acids, although other longer forms of the neurohormone are found (e.g., somatostatin-28). Somatostatinergic cells run from the paraventricular nucleus of the hypothalamus to the median eminence. The wide distribution of somatostatinergic activity throughout the body is shown in Fig. 11, and the various physiologic effects are outlined in Fig. 12. GHRH and somatostatin appear to have an antagonistic role in the control of GH release from the anterior pituitary. The secretion of GH is dependent, therefore, on the balance between the stimulatory action of GHRH, and the inhibitory action of somatostatin. As this balance shifts to-and-fro, GH is secreted in a pulsatile and rhythmic manner.

The feedback control loops for GHRH in GH secretion are shown in Figs. 13 and 14. The short loop feeds back to the hypothalamus and inhibits GHRH at the genomic level, while stimulating somatostatin. The long loop involves inhibitory feedback of peripheral IGF-I on GH release and reciprocal stimulation of somatostatin secretion.

Hormonal Regulation of GH Secretion

Glucocorticoids inhibit GHRH-induced GH secretion, either via a direct action on GH-secreting cells or by increasing the inhibitory action of somatostatin (14). Patients with hypocortisolism have low GH levels, and this condition is reversed by the administration of exogenous glucocorticoids. Because glucocorticoids also increase GH gene transcription (15,16), they probably play a dual regulatory role, depending on whether administration is chronic or acute. Thyroid hormones are important regulators of linear growth, and hypothyroidism is associated with decreased GH secretion and decreased dynamic responses (17,18). Replacement of thyroid hormones restores normal GH secretion and responses (19). It is believed that GHRH action is impaired by thyroid hormone deficiency, although it is not known if this is a genomic or a receptor-based action. Hyperthyroidism is also associated with impaired stimulated GH secretion, although a rise in GH pulse fre-

---

Anatomic distribution of somatostatin

- Central nervous system
- Peripheral nervous system – broadly distributed in fibers
  - Genitourinary
  - Heart
  - Eye
  - Thyroid
  - Thymus
  - Skin
  - Intestinal myenteric neurons
- Pancreatic islet D cells
- Gastric and intestinal epithelium
- Salivary glands
- Parafollicular cells of thyroid

FIG. 11. Anatomic distribution of somatostatin.

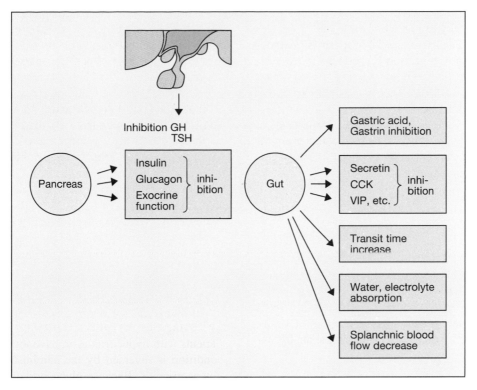

FIG. 12. Inhibitory and regulatory effects of somatostatin.

quency has also been noted in this condition. Casanueva (20) has suggested that thyroid hormones may have a bimodal action, inhibiting GHRH while at the same time decreasing somatostatin release from the hypothalamus.

Gonadal hormones may regulate GH secretion in a sexually dimorphic manner, probably interacting with the balance of GHRH and somatostatin release from the hypothalamus (21). Estradiol may influence the control of hypothalamic somatostatin levels via an effect on catecholamines. It is also believed that estradiol alters α_2-adrenoreceptor activity, which also regulates the activity of somatostatinergic neural activity (22). This inhibition of somatostatin release may largely explain the higher circulating GH levels observed in premenopausal women. The role of testosterone in GH regulation is unclear, although it may stimulate somatostatinergic tone.

Metabolic Regulation of GH Secretion

Physiologic variations in metabolic requirements and supplies are known to have an important regulatory action for GH secretion. Hyperglycemia after ingestion of an oral glucose load suppresses GH release in normal individuals, and failure of oral glucose to suppress GH is a standard test used in the diagnosis of acromegaly. Hypoglycemia, whether constitutional or insulin-induced, stimulates GH secretion (23). It appears that the absolute level of intracellular glucose rather than the rate of decrease of glucose concentration is the primary hypoglycemic stimulator of GH release (24), although this remains a subject of controversy. In addition to carbohydrate metabolism, alterations in protein and lipid metabolism also affect GH release. Elevation in the concentration of plasma free fatty acid is a profound inhibitor of GH secretion, whereas GH secretion is stimulated by decreased free fatty acid levels (25,26). It is probable that the mechanism of action is via an effect on somatostatinergic tone rather than by affecting GHRH or the pituitary directly. Amino acid uptake in peripheral tissues is promoted by GH (27), and experimental administration of amino acids stimulates GH secretion (28). Once again, it is believed that amino acids act on the hypothalamus at the level of inhibition of somatostatin release.

Neurologic Regulation of GH Secretion

The neurologic control of GH secretion is complex, and a full discussion of the interplay of separate neurologic sys-

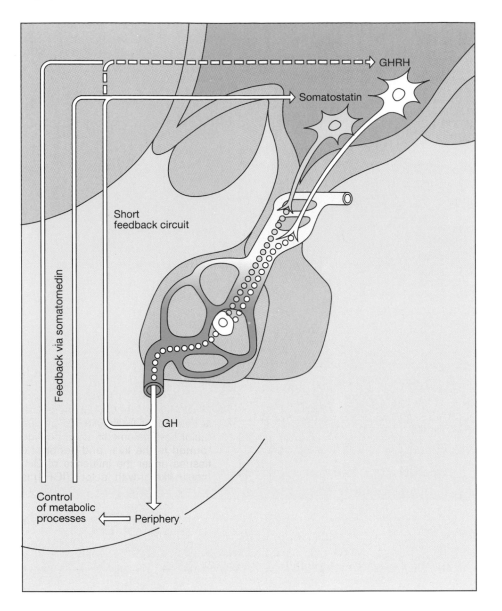

FIG. 13. Regulation of GH secretion. The secretion of GH is stimulated by GHRH and is inhibited by somatostatin release from the hypothalamus.

tems and the hypothalamic–pituitary axis is beyond the scope of this book. A comprehensive review of the neuroendocrine regulation of growth hormone has been published by Bertherat and colleagues (29).

Adrenergic, cholinergic, GABAergic (30), and many other neural systems (e.g., opioid, galanin, serotonin) have been shown to modulate hypothalamic GHRH and somatostatin release. Adrenergic neurons regulate GH secretion by inhibiting somatostatin release (31,32) and by altering the pulsatility of GH secretion (33). Cholinergic neurons appear to be intimately involved in promoting GH secretion during activity and sleep, probably via inhibition of hypothalamic somatostatinergic tone (34). In their review, Bertherat et al. (29) suggest that galanin-containing neurons may enhance GH secretion by stimulating GHRH and inhibiting somatostatin.

GROWTH HORMONE BINDING PROTEIN

Approximately 30% of circulating GH is carried bound to a high-affinity GH binding protein (GHBP), first described in the mid-1980s (35–37). It appears that GHBP is structurally very similar to the extracellular portion of the GH receptor, and both the GH receptor and GHBP may be derived from the same mRNA source (38). A concise review of GH receptor function is provided in a recent report by Postel-Vinay and Finidori (39). GHBP levels as measured by radioimmunoassay (RIA) are decreased in acromegalic patients (40). Treatment with the somatostatin analogue octreotide leads to a rise in GHBP levels (41), and GHBP measurements may therefore represent a new tool for the diagnosis of acromegaly.

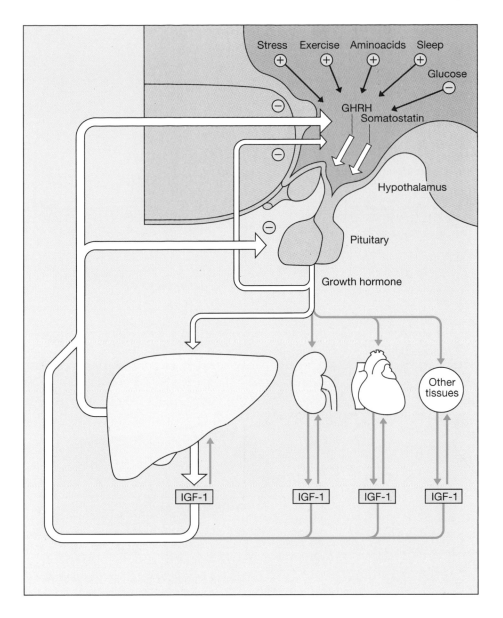

FIG. 14. The stimulatory effect of GHRH on pituitary GH secretion is modulated by insulin-like growth factor I (somatomedin C), a peptide formed in the liver and peripheral tissues under the influence of GH. Insulin-like growth factor I (IGF-I) is thus involved in the negative feedback loop governing GH secretion. GH secretion is stimulated by stress, exercise and protein and inhibited by glucose. Dark lines, peripheral to central regulation; open lines, central regulation; light lines, putative regulation.

INSULIN-LIKE GROWTH FACTOR-I

Structure, Synthesis, and Secretion

As described above, GH is secreted by the pituitary under the control of the hypothalamic hormones GHRH and somatostatin and of other hormonal, metabolic, and neurologic factors. However, GH is not directly responsible for many growth-promoting effects. Instead, GH causes the release of insulin-like growth factors (IGFs), also termed somatomedins (Fig. 15). These factors, IGF-I (42) and IGF-II (43), were characterized in the late 1970s [although IGF-I activity had been discovered 20 years earlier (44)], and they received their name because they exhibit structural similarity to proinsulin. IGF-I is a 70–amino-acid single-chain protein that is of primary interest in acromegaly

because it is closely regulated by GH secretion (45). IGF-I concentrations rise during puberty (46,47) and correlate well with GH receptor activity in the liver. Many tissues, such as bone and skeletal muscle, release IGF-I in response to GH, but the majority of IGF-I synthesis occurs in the liver.

Two IGF receptors exist: type 1, which has high affinity for IGF-I and IGF-II, and type 2, which has high affinity for IGF-II and lower affinity for IGF-I (48,49). The signal transduction mechanisms for IGF receptor interactions are complex and are incompletely understood at this time. It appears that GH acts both on liver cells to produce IGF-I (which then circulates to distant sites and stimulates growth), and also stimulates local IGF-I production in tissues such as cartilage and bone. In a comprehensive review of GH and IGF-I effects, Daughaday (50) suggests that

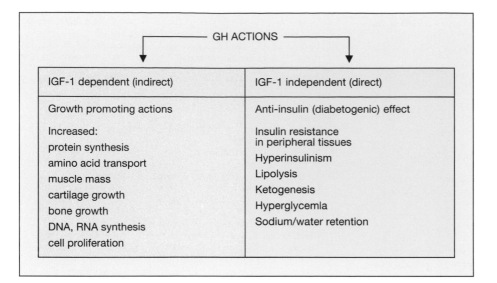

FIG. 15. Physiologic actions of growth hormone.

both of these mechanisms exist in parallel. Laboratory studies have demonstrated that IGF-I administration causes increases in skeletal and organ growth in hypophysectomized and transgenic animals (51,52). IGF-I levels are increased in acromegaly and reliably reflect integrated 24-h GH secretion (53), which provides the clinician with an excellent confirmatory test in suspected acromegaly, as well as a marker for disease activity during and after treatment.

Insulin-Like Growth Factor Binding Proteins

Insulin-like growth factor binding proteins (IGFBPs) were first isolated and characterized during the mid-1980s, and it now appears that there are six IGFBPs, which bind IGF-I and IGF-II. The association of IGFs with their binding proteins is regulated by a complex system of proteases and receptors [for reviews see Zapf (54) and Shimasaki et al. (55)]. All IGFBPs bind IGF-I and IGF-II with high affinity, although insulin, which has the same three-dimensional structure as IGF-I, does not interfere with binding kinetics (56). Importantly, IGFBPs regulate circulating IGF-I levels and therefore are significant modulators of IGF-I activity in normal and acromegalic individuals. Zapf et al. (54) reported that IGFBPs are present in the serum as two large complexes of 150 kDa and 40–50 kDa. Only IGFBP-3 is found as part of the vital 150-kDa ternary compound, and it appears that IGFBP-3 is the predominant IGFBP regulator of serum IGF-I binding. In acromegaly, IGFBP-3 has been the subject of much recent interest because it is GH- (and probably IGF-I)-dependent. Grinspoon et al. (57) have suggested that IGFBP-3 can be used as a sensitive biochemical marker for elevated GH in suspected cases of acromegaly, although de Herder et al. (58) have noted that IGFBP-3 has no additional discriminatory value over IGF-I in the assessment of disease activity in

acromegaly. Somatostatin (59) and its analogues octreotide (60) and lanreotide (61) have been shown to stimulate IGFBP-1, and it may be that these drugs mediate their clinical actions partially by altering IGFBP concentration (62). The dopamine agonist bromocriptine has no such effect on IGFBP-1 secretion (63).

REFERENCES

1. Stolar MW, Amburn K, Baumann G. Plasma "big" and "big-big" growth hormone (GH) in man: an oligomeric series composed of structurally diverse GH monomers. *J Clin Endocrinol Metab* 1984;59:212–8.
2. Owerbach D, Martial JA, Baxter JD, Rutter WJ, Shows TB. Genes for growth hormone, chorionic somatomammotropin and a growth hormone-like gene are located on chromosome 17 in humans. *Science* 1980;209:289.
3. Cryer PE, Daughaday WH. Growth hormone. In: Martini L, Besser GM, eds. *Clinical neuroendocrinology.* New York: Academic Press, 1977:243–7.
4. Scippo ML, Frankenne F, Van Beeuman J, Igout A, Hennen G. Human placental growth hormone: proof of identity with the GH-V gene product by N-terminal microsequence analysis. *Arch in Physiol Biochim* 1989;97:B59.
5. Hennen G, Frankenne F, Closset J, et al. A human placental GH: increasing levels during second half of pregnancy with pituitary GH suppression as revealed by monoclonal antibody radioimmunoassays. *Int J Fertil* 1985;30:27.
6. Beckers A, Stevenaert A, Foidart JM, Hennen G, Frankenne F. Placental and pituitary growth hormone secretion during pregnancy in acromegalic women. *J Clin Endocrinol Metab* 1990;71:725–31.
7. Mendelson WB. Studies of human growth hormone secretion in sleep and waking. *Int Rev Neurobiol* 1982;23:367–89.
8. Casanueva FF, Villanueva L, Cabranes JA, Cabezas-Cerrato J, Fernandez-Cruz A. Cholinergic mediation of growth hormone secretion elicited by arginine, clonidine and physical exercise in man. *J Clin Endocrinol Metab* 1984;59:526–30.
9. Plotnick LP, Thompson RG, Kowarski A, DeLacerda L, Migeon CJ, Blizzard RM. Circadian variation of integrated concentration of growth hormone in children and adults. *J Clin Endocrinol Metab* 1975;40:240–7.
10. Ho KY, Evans WS, Blizzard RM, et al. Effects of sex and age on the 24-hour profile of growth hormone secretion in man: importance of endogenous estradiol concentrations. *J Clin Endocrinol Metab* 1987; 64:51–8.

11. Schaeffer F, Baumann G, Haffner D, et al. Multifactorial control of the elimination kinetics of unbound (free) growth hormone (GH) in the human: regulation by age, adiposity, renal function and steady state concentrations of GH in plasma. *J Clin Endocrinol Metab* 1996; 81:22–31.
12. Guillemin R, Brazeau P, Bohlen P, et al. Growth hormone-releasing factor from a human pancreatic tumor that caused acromegaly. *Science* 1982;218:585.
13. Casanueva FF. Physiology of growth hormone secretion and action. *Endocrine Metab Clin North Am* 1992;21:483–517.
14. Casanueva FF, Burguera B, Tome MA, et al. Depending on the time of administration, dexamethasone potentiates or blocks growth hormone releasing hormone-induced growth hormone release in man. *Neuroendocrinology* 1988;47:46.
15. Martial JA, Seeburg PH, Guenzi D, et al. Regulation of growth hormone gene expression: Synergistic effects of thyroid and glucocorticoid hormones. *Proc Natl Acad Sci USA* 1977;74:4293.
16. Karin M, Castrillo JL, Theill LE. Growth hormone gene regulation: a paradigm for cell-type specific gene activation. *Trends Genet* 1990; 6:92–6.
17. Valcavi R, Dieguez C, Zini M, et al. Effect of pyridostigmine and pirenzepine on GH responses to GHRH in hyperthyroid patients. *Clin Endocrinol* 1991;35:141.
18. Finkelstein JW, Boyar RM, Hellman L. Growth hormone secretion in hypothyroidism. *J Clin Endocrinol Metab* 1974;38:634.
19. Williams T, Maxon H, Thorner MO, et al. Blunted growth hormone (GH) response to GH-releasing hormone in hypothyroidism resolves in the euthyroid state. *J Clin Endocrinol Metab* 1985;61:454.
20. Casanueva FF. Physiology of growth hormone secretion and action. *Endocrine Metab Clin North Am* 1992;21:483–517.
21. Devesa J, Lois N, Arce V, Diaz MJ, Lima L, Tresguerres JAF. The role of sexual steroids in the modulation of growth hormone (GH) secretion in humans. *J Steroid Biochem Mol Biol* 1991;40:165–73.
22. Devesa J, Arce V, Lois N, Tresguerres JAF, Lima L. α2-Adrenergic agonism enhances the growth hormone (GH) response to GH-releasing hormone through an inhibition of hypothalamic somatostatin release in normal men. *J Clin Endocrinol Metab* 1990;71:1518–88.
23. Roth J, Glick SM, Yalow RS, et al. Hypoglycemia: a potent stimulus of growth hormone. *Science* 1963;140:987.
24. Amiel SA, Simonson DC, Tamborlane WV, et al. Rate of glucose fall does not affect counterregulatory hormone responses to hypoglycemia in normal and diabetic subjects. *Diabetes* 1987;36:518.
25. Imaki T, Shibaski T, Shizume K, et al. The effect of free fatty acids on growth hormone releasing hormone mediated GH secretion in man. *J Clin Endocrinol Metab* 1985;60:290.
26. Irie M, Sakuma M, Tsushima M, et al. Effect of nicotinic acid administration on plasma growth hormone concentrations. *Proc Soc Exp Biol Med* 1967;126:708.
27. Knobil E, Wolf RC, Greep RO, Wilhelmi AE. Effect of a primate growth hormone preparation on nitrogen metabolism in the hypophysectomized rhesus monkey. *Endocrinology* 1957;60:166.
28. Merrimee TJ, Lillicrap DA, Rabinowitz D. Effect of arginine on serum levels of human growth hormone. *Lancet* 1965;2:668.
29. Bertherat J, Bluet-Pajot MT, Epelbaum J. Neuroendocrine regulation of growth hormone. *Eur J Endocrinol* 1995;132:12–24.
30. Rage F, Benyassi A, Arancibia S, Tapia Arancibia L. GABA-glutamate interaction in the control of somatostatin from hypothalamic neurons in primary culture: in vivo corroboration. *Endocrinology* 1992;130:1056–62.
31. Devesa J, Diaz MJ, Tresguerres JAF, Arce V, Lima L. Evidence that α2-adrenergic pathways play a major role in growth hormone (GH) neuroregulation. *J Clin Endocrinol Metab* 1991;73:251–6.
32. Devesa J, Arce V, Lois N, Tresguerres JAF, Lima L. α2-Adrenergic agonism enhances the growth hormone (GH) response to GH-releasing hormone through an inhibition of hypothalamic somatostatin release in normal men. *J Clin Endocrinol Metab* 1990;71:1518–88.
33. Bluet-Pajot MT, Bertherat J, Epelbaum J, Kordon C. Neural and pituitary mechanisms involved in growth hormone regulation. *J Pediatr Res* 1993;6:357–69.
34. Casanueva FF, Villanueva L, Cabranes JA, Cabezas-Cerrato J, Fernandz-Cruz A. Cholinergic mediation of growth hormone secretion elicited by arginine, clonidine and physical exercise in man. *J Clin Endocrinol Metab* 1984;59:526–30.
35. Baumann G, Stolar M, Amburn K, Barsano CP, DeVries BC. A specific growth hormone-binding protein in human plasma: initial characterization. *J Clin Endocrinol Metab* 1986;62:134–41.
36. Herrington AC, Ymer S, Stevenson J. Identification and characterization of specific binding proteins for growth hormone in normal human sera. *J Clin Invest* 1986;77:1817–23.
37. Ymer SI, Herrington AC. Evidence for the specific binding of growth hormone to a receptor-like protein in rabbit serum. *Mol Cell Endocrinol* 1985;41:153.
38. Leung DW, Spencer SA, Cachianes G, et al. Growth hormone receptor and serum binding protein: purification, cloning and expression. *Nature* 1987;330:537–43.
39. Postel-Vinay MC, Finidori J. Growth hormone receptor: structure and signal transduction. *Eur J Endocrinol* 1995;133:654–9.
40. Kratzsch J, Blum WF, Ventz M, Selisko T, Birkenmeyer G, Keller E. Growth hormone binding protein-related immunoreactivity in the serum of patients with acromegaly is regulated inversely by growth hormone concentration. *Eur J Endocrinol* 1995;132:306–12.
41. Roelen CAM, Donker GH, Thijssen JHH, Koppeschaar HPF, Blankenstein MA. High affinity growth hormone binding protein in plasma of patients with acromegaly and the effect of octreotide treatment. *Clin Endocrinol* 1991;37:373–8.
42. Riderknecht E, Humbel RE. The amino acid sequence of human insulin-like growth factor I and its structural homology with proinsulin. *J Biol Chem* 1978;253:2769.
43. Riderknecht E, Humbel RE. Primary structure of human insulin-like growth factor II. *FEBS Lett* 1978;89:283.
44. Salmon WD, Daughaday WH. A hormonally controlled serum factor which stimulates sulfate incorporation by cartilage in vitro. *J Lab Clin Med* 1957;49:825.
45. Matthews LS, Norstedt G, Palmiter RG. Regulation of insulin-like growth factor-I gene expression by GH. *Proc Natl Acad Sci USA* 1986;83:9343–7.
46. Silbergeld A, Litwin A, Bruchis S, et al. Insulin-like growth factor I (IGF-I) in healthy children, adolescents and adults as determined by a radioimmunoassay specific for the synthetic 53-70 peptide region. *Clin Endocrinol* 1986;25:67.
47. Hall K, Sara VR. Somatomedin levels in childhood, adolescence and in adult life. *Clin Endocrinol* 1984;13:91–112.
48. Neely EK, Beukers MW, Oh Y, et al. Insulin-like growth factor receptors. *Acta Paediatr Scand* 1991;372:116.
49. Morgan DO, Edman JC, Standring DN, et al. Insulin-like growth factor 2 receptor as a multifunctional binding protein. *Nature* 1987; 329:301.
50. Daughaday WE. A personal history of the origin of the somatomedin hypothesis and recent challenges to its validity. *Perspect Biol Med* 1989;32:194.
51. Matthews LS, Hammer RE, Behringer RR, et al. Insulin-like growth factor I stimulates growth in hypophysectomized rats. *Nature* 1982;296:252.
52. Behringer RR, Lewin TM, Quaife CJ, et al. Expression of insulin-like growth factor I stimulates normal somatic growth in growth hormone-deficient transgenic mice. *Endocrinology* 1990;127:1033.
53. Clemmons DR, VanWyk JJ, Ridgway EC, et al. Evaluation of acromegaly by radioimmunoassay of somatomedin C. *N Engl J Med* 1979;301:1138–42.
54. Zapf J. Physiological role of the insulin-like growth factor binding proteins. *Eur J Endocrinol* 1995;132:645–54.
55. Shimasaki S, Ling N. Identification and molecular characterization of insulin-like growth factor binding proteins (IGFBP-1, -2, -3, -4, -5, -6). *Prog Growth Factor Res* 1991;3:243–66.
56. Rechler MM. Insulin-like growth factor binding proteins. *Vitam Horm NY* 1993;47:1–114.
57. Grinspoon S, Clemmons D, Swearingen B, Klibanski A. Serum insulin-like growth factor binding protein-3 levels in the diagnosis of acromegaly. *J Clin Endocrinol Metab* 1995;80:927–32.
58. deHerder WW, van der Lely AJ, Janssen JAMJL, Uitterlinden P, Hofland LJ, Lamberts SWJ. IGFBP-3 is a poor parameter for assessment of clinical activity in acromegaly. *Clin Endocrinol* 1995; 43:501–5.
59. Ørskov H, Wolthers T, Grøfte T, Flyvbjerg A, Vilstrup H, Hamburg O. Somatostatin-stimulated insulin-like growth factor binding protein-1 release is abolished by hyperinsulinemia. *J Clin Endocrinol Metab* 1994;78:138–40.

60. Ezzat S, Ren S-G, Braunstein GD, Melmed S. Octreotide stimulates insulin-like growth factor binding protein-1: a potential pituitary-independent mechanism for drug action. *J Clin Endocrinol Metab* 1992;75:1459–63.
61. Wolthers T, Grøfte T, Flyvbjerg A, et al. Dose-dependent stimulation of insulin-like growth factor binding protein-1 by Lanreotide, a somatostatin analog. *J Clin Endocrinol Metab* 1994;78:141–4.
62. Melmed S. Octreotide stimulates insulin-like growth factor binding protein-1: a novel mechanism of drug action on acromegaly. *Semin Oncol* 1994;21(Suppl 13):65–9.
63. deHerder W, Uitterlinden P, van der Lely AJ, Hofland LJ, Lamberts SWJ. Octreotide, but not bromocriptine, increases circulating insulin-like growth factor binding protein-1 levels in acromegaly. *Eur J Endocrinol* 1995;133:195–9.

CHAPTER 3

Acromegaly: Epidemiology, Etiology, and Classification

EPIDEMIOLOGY

The most recent estimates of the prevalence of acromegaly are approximately 55 patients per million population in the Newcastle area (U.K.) (1), 69 patients per million population in the Göteborg area (Sweden) (2), 63 patients per million population in Northern Ireland (3), and 60 patients per million population in Spain (4) (Table 1). The incidence was calculated in these studies to be approximately three to four new cases per million population per year. Since the population of the United States is over 250 million, it can be estimated that around 750–1,000 new cases of acromegaly occur in the United States each year. All epidemiologic studies have shown that the frequency of acromegaly is the same in both sexes.

Age at Onset and Diagnosis

In a series of 256 acromegalic patients collated by Nabarro (5), the mean age at onset in men was 32.7 years (range 8–62 years) and in women 34.9 years (range 9–64 years), whereas the mean age at diagnosis was 42.3 years for men (range 15–82 years) and 43.8 years for women (range 14–73 years). Rajasoorya et al. (6) estimated the

duration of symptoms before diagnosis as 7 years and the mean age at diagnosis as 41 years. A similar age pattern was reported by Harris et al. (7) in a series of 178 acromegalic patients. All of these results were confirmed by the largest epidemiologic study of acromegaly, involving 500 patients, published by Ezzat et al. (8) (Fig. 16). Younger patients tend to harbor more aggressive tumors with prominent clinical changes, whereas older patients may develop symptoms insidiously over many years. This insidious course often results in a considerable time lag (7–10 years) between the onset of acromegaly and the diagnosis (Fig. 17).

Prognosis

The prognosis for acromegaly is highly dependent on early detection and treatment of the disease. Acromegalic patients demonstrate a two- to fourfold increase in mortali-

TABLE 1. Incidence and prevalence of acromegaly from epidemiological studies		
Reference	Prevalence (per million population)	Incidence (per million population)
Alexander et al. (1)	38	2.8
Bengtsson et al. (2)	69	3.3
Ritchie et al. (3)	63	4.0
Extabe et al. (4)	60	3.1

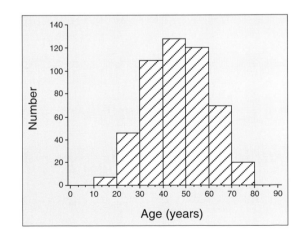

FIG. 16. Age distribution by decades of 500 patients with acromegaly. (From Ezzat S, Forster MJ, Berchtold P, Harris AG. Acromegaly. Clinical and biochemical features in 500 patients. *Medicine* 1994;73:233–40.)

	Delay in diagnosis					
	Male		Female		Combined	
Age at diagnosis (years)	Mean delay (years)	Number	Mean delay (years)	Number	Mean delay (years)	Number
Under 31	6.8	28	5.2	30	6.0	58
31-40	7.9	38	6.1	22	7.2	60
41-50	8.9	32	11.9	24	10.2	56
Over 50	12.6	35	12.1	47	12.3	82
All ages	9.1	133	9.3	123	9.2	256

FIG. 17. Relationship between delay in diagnosis and age of patients. [From J.D.N. Nabarro, 1987 (5).]

ty relative to the general population. Recently, Bates et al. (9) reported an overall mortality rate of 2.63 compared with the general population. Of the 194 patients reviewed by Wright et al. (10), 26% of the deaths occurred before the age of 50 years and 64% by the age of 60. Rajasoorya et al. (6) reported that acromegalic patients demonstrated a three-fold increased mortality from cardiovascular disease and were at 3.3-fold higher risk for death from cerebrovascular disease. The mortality rates in acromegaly from vascular, respiratory, and malignant causes are shown in Fig. 18. The mean age at death as determined by the above epidemiologic studies ranges from 57 to 64 years, which underscores the significant effects of acromegaly on the life span.

Treatment of acromegaly extends the promise of improved quality of life and possible extended life expectancy for these patients, although more formal outcome studies are required. An indication of this comes from the study by Bates et al. (9). When patients with a lowest measured GH level of <5 μg/L were assessed alone, they had a mortality rate of 2.01, and those with GH levels of <2.5 μg/L had an even lower mortality rate of 1.42, which does not represent any statistical difference from the general population. Furthermore, Rajasoorya and colleagues (6) found that reduced

survival in acromegaly was significantly associated with a high post-treatment GH level. These results indicate that good long-term suppression of GH levels may have a highly beneficial effect on the life expectancy of acromegalic patients.

Symptoms at presentation usually include acral enlargement, coarsening of facial features, profuse sweating, carpal tunnel syndrome, headache, and osteoarthritis. However, in the series reported by Nabarro (5), only 13% of patients actively sought medical attention for changes in appearance (coarsening of facial features, soft-tissue swelling) or enlargement of extremities (bony proliferation), thus underscoring the elusiveness of these symptoms. The signs and symptoms at presentation from 500 acromegalic patients are shown in Fig. 19.

ETIOLOGY OF ACROMEGALY

Hypothalamic and Pituitary Lesions

In the vast majority of cases (ca. 95%), acromegaly is caused by excessive secretion of GH from cells of the anterior pituitary (11) (Fig. 20). The precise etiology of this hypersecretion is still a matter of debate. The more persuasive view is that acromegaly arises from an intrinsic defect within the pituitary gland, resulting in the development of an adenoma which thereafter functions autonomously (12). In support of this explanation, approximately 40% of all pituitary adenomas have a monoclonal origin, indicating that the tumor arises from a mutation in a single cell (13). The gene believed to be responsible encodes the production of a Gs-protein α-subchain, which mediates receptor-based hormonal signaling (14–16). It appears that two specific amino acid substitutions can lead to the G-protein abnormality (Arg 201 or Gln 227) that causes GH hypersecretion. Because this gene has also been implicated in other endocrine-active tumors, it has been termed an oncogene, named *gsp*. [For a recent review see Melmed et al. (17).] In addition, complete surgical removal of a well-circumscribed GH-producing adenoma can be curative, indicating that in many cases the disease is of purely pituitary origin.

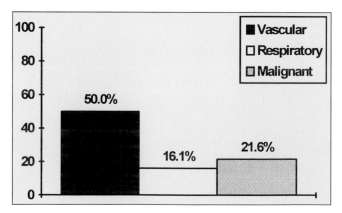

FIG. 18. Data derived from seven major epidemiological and outcome studies in acromegaly (1–4,6,9,10). Respiratory causes of death were not reported in three of the studies used, while deaths due to vascular and malignant causes were reported in all seven.

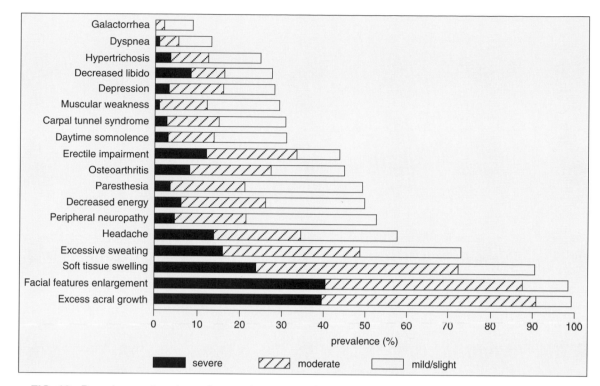

FIG. 19. Prevalence of various signs and symptoms in 500 patients with acromegaly. Severe features are represented by histograms, moderate by diagonally hatched, and mild/slight features by open histograms. (From Ezzat S, Forster MJ, Berchtold P, Harris AG. Acromegaly. Clinical and biochemical features in 500 patients. *Medicine* 1994;73:233–40.)

According to a second hypothesis, the primary dysfunction in acromegaly originates as a hypothalamic hormonal imbalance (either hypersecretion of GHRH or hyposecretion of somatostatin) (see Fig. 20). Overproduction of GHRH by functional hypothalamic tumors, such as hamartomas, choristomas, gliomas, and gangliocytomas, can cause acromegaly by inducing proliferation of GH-secreting pituitary cells. Although such GHRH release constitutes a major part of the pathophysiologic mechanism in ectopic acromegaly (see below), it is not known whether abnormal hypothalamic secretion can induce the formation of a pituitary adenoma. Riedel and colleagues (18) noted that GH pulse generation was independent of GHRH levels in many patients, and Attanasio et al. (19) recently noted that somatostatinergic tone does not appear to fluctuate in acromegaly.

In summary, it is possible that as data from future basic and clinical research accumulate, an integrated evaluation of the pathogenesis of acromegaly involving both hypothalamic and pituitary factors in pituitary tumorigenesis may evolve.

Ectopic Lesions

A variety of ectopic lesions (bronchial or intestinal carcinoids, pancreatic islet cell carcinomas, or pheochromocytomas), which produce GHRH, are a rare cause of acromegaly (1%). [For in-depth reviews see Faglia et al. (20) and Melmed and Rushakoff (21).] These tumors lead to somatotroph hyperplasia, GH hypersecretion, and therefore to acromegaly. Pure ectopic GH-secreting tumors are extremely rare, and to date only one has been reported in the world literature (22).

CLASSIFICATION OF GH-SECRETING PITUITARY ADENOMAS

GH-secreting pituitary adenomas can be classified according to staining affinities of the cellular cytoplasm, growth pattern, endocrine activity, histologic appearance, electron microscopic features, granularity of cytoplasm, cellular composition, and cytogenesis (Figs. 21 and 22).

Histopathologic Classification

Kovacs and Horvath (23) developed the following classification of pituitary GH-secreting adenomas:

Densely granulated GH-producing cell adenoma.
Sparsely granulated GH-producing cell adenoma.
Mixed GH- and prolactin-producing cell adenoma.

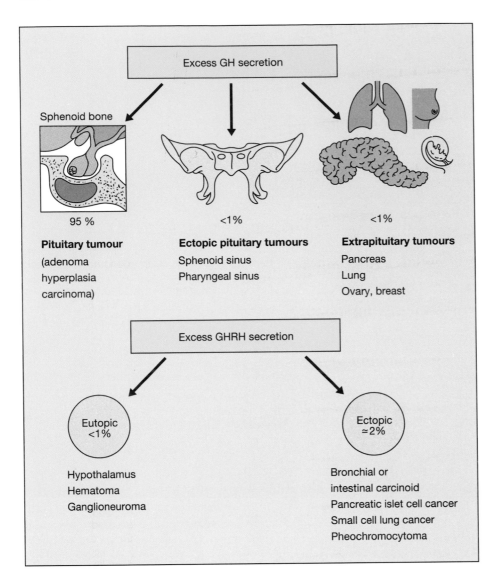

FIG. 20. Pathogenesis of acromegaly. [Adapted from S. Melmed, 1990 (11).]

Acidophilic stem-cell adenoma.
Somatomammotrope adenoma.
Growth hormone cell carcinoma.
Plurihormonal adenoma (secreting prolactin and/or thyroid-
   stimulating hormone).

The first two types (densely and sparsely granulated) are
the most common in acromegaly.

Receptor Classification

Biochemical studies of excised acromegalic tumor tissue
have shown that it often contains receptors for the various
hypothalamic releasing factors, notably somatostatin (24).
Immense advances in the field of somatostatin receptor
research have been made during the past few years. Five

somatostatin receptors have been characterized, all of
which belong to the G-protein family of receptors, with
seven membrane-spanning areas [for a review of the molecular pharmacology of somatostatin receptors see Bruns et
al. (25)]. These receptors are distributed throughout many
tissues, especially on endocrine-active cells. The binding
characteristics of the somatostatin receptor subtypes differ,
indicating a variation in functions subserved by each subtype across various organ systems.

The main receptor subpopulations found in pituitary adenomas are types 1, 2 and 5 (26), and the expression of certain receptor populations may vary with adenoma cell characteristics (27). Because these receptors are known to be
functional, their presence probably plays a major role in the
medical treatment of such tumors with a long-acting
somatostatin analogue, such as octreotide. In parallel with
basic research, a new avenue has opened up in nuclear

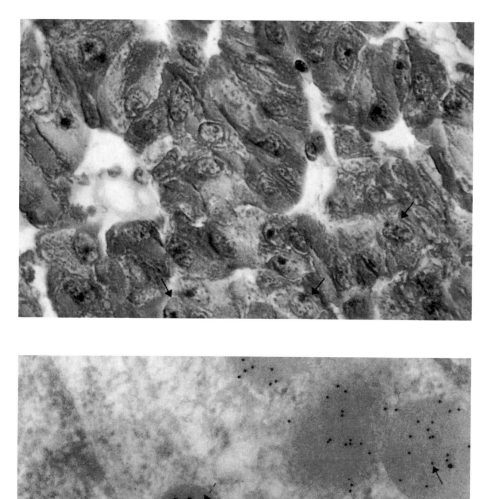

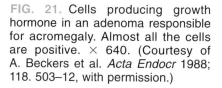

FIG. 21. Cells producing growth hormone in an adenoma responsible for acromegaly. Almost all the cells are positive. × 640. (Courtesy of A. Beckers et al. *Acta Endocr* 1988; 118. 503–12, with permission.)

FIG. 22. Mixed pituitary adenoma (GH–PRL) as revealed by electron microscopy double gold immunostaining of GH (→) cells (gold particle 10 nm) and of PRL (→) cells (gold particle 15 nm) and of a mixed cell synthesizing both GH and PRL. In this case the two hormones are produced by different cell populations. × 86,000. (Courtesy of A. Beckers et al. *Acta Endocr* 1988; 118:503–12, with permission.)

medicine with the advent of radiolabeled somatostatin scintigraphy. This has enabled clinicians to identify tumor loci by their somatostatin receptor positivity (Fig. 23). It has been suggested that the demonstration of somatostatin receptor positivity may be used to predict responsiveness to octreotide treatment (28). Dopamine and thyrotropin-releasing hormone receptors have also been demonstrated in pituitary tumors, although this observation has not been used in a formal classification system, provocation tests using L-dopa and TRH have been used diagnostically in acromegaly research.

Radioanatomic Classification

Vezina and Maltais (29) developed a size-based anatomic classification of pituitary adenomas based on radiotomograms of the skull (groups 0–IV). Furthermore, a system for the staging of suprasellar extension and invasive properties (stages A–C) of pituitary tumors was devised by Guiot et al. (30), based on pneumoencephalograms of the pituitary region. More recently, stages D and E were added to describe lateral tumor extensions based on CT scans of the pituitary. These various classification systems are represented graphically in Fig. 24.

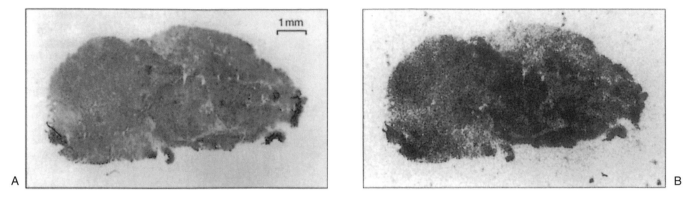

FIG. 23. Somatostatin receptors in a growth-hormone producing pituitary adenoma. **(A)** A hematoxylin-stained section and **(B)** the corresponding autoradiogram. (Courtesy of J.-C. Reubi, University of Berne, Switzerland.)

Sella turcica (bony contours)	Floor	Pituitary adenoma	Grades of sella turcica enlargement	EXTRASELLAR EXTENSIONS				
				Suprasellar (symmetrical)			Parasellar (asymmetrical)	
				A	B	C	D	E
Normal	Intact		0					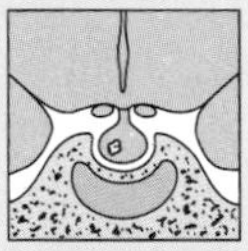 (according to Wilson)
Not enlarged	May be eroded	Enclosed micro-adenoma (<10 mm)	I	Filling the chiasmatic cistern (10 mm)	Elevating the recesses of the third ventricle (20 mm)			
Enlarged	Intact	Enclosed macro-adenoma (>10 mm)	II			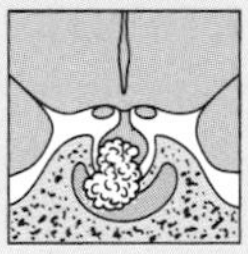 Filling the anterior third ventricle (>30 mm) 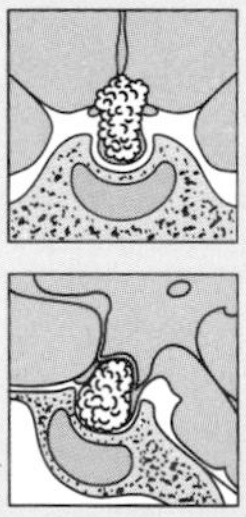	Intracranial extensions (frontal, temporal or posterior fossa) 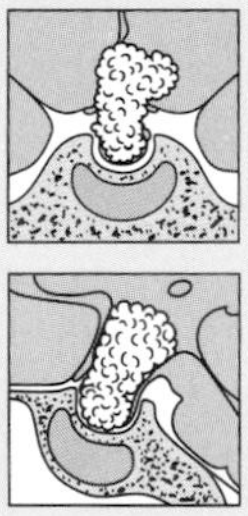	Extracranial lateral extension toward cavernous sinus 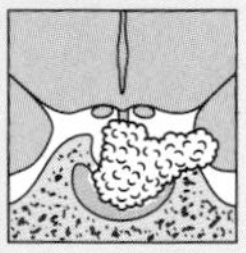
Enlarged	Eroded	Invasive macro-adenoma	III					
Enlarged	Diffusely eroded	Invasive macro-adenoma	IV 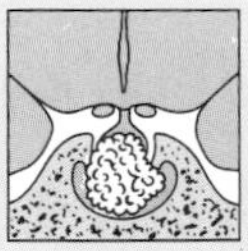					

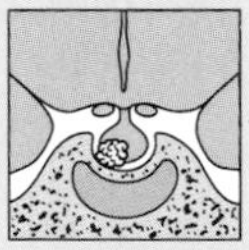

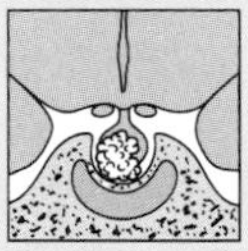

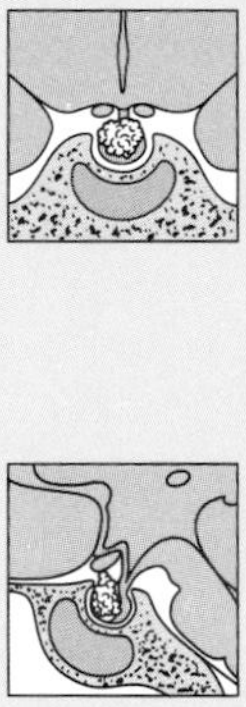

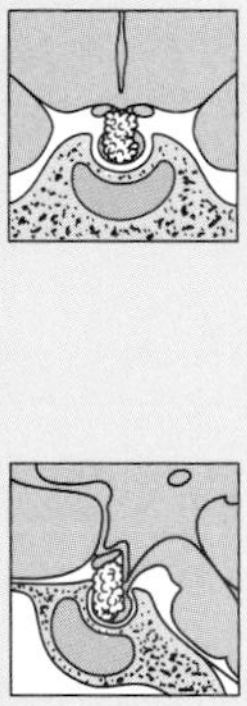

FIG. 24. Radioanatomical classification of GH-secreting pituitary adenomas. (Based on CT-MRI according to Guiot, Vezina, Hardy, and Wilson.)

REFERENCES

1. Alexander L, Appleton D, Hall R, Ross WM, Wilkinson R. Epidemiology of acromegaly in the Newcastle region. *Clin Endocrinol* 1980;12:71–9.
2. Bengtsson BÅ, Eden S, Ernest I, Oden A, Sjögren B. Epidemiology and long term survival in acromegaly. *Acta Med Scand* 1988;223:327–35.
3. Ritchie CM, Atkinson AB, Kennedy AL, et al. Ascertainment and natural history of treated acromegaly in Northern Ireland. *Ulster Med J* 1990;59:55–62.
4. Extabe J, Gaztambide S, Latorre P, Vazquez J. Acromegaly: an epidemiological study. *J Endocrinol Invest* 1993;16:181–7.
5. Nabarro JDN. Acromegaly. *Clin Endocrinol* 1987;26:481–512.
6. Rajasoorya C, Holdaway IM, Wrightson P, Scott DJ, Ibbertson HK. Determinants of clinical outcome and survival in acromegaly. *Clin Endocrinol* 1994;41:95–102.
7. Harris AG, Prestele H, Herold K, Boerlin V. Long-term efficacy of Sandostatin (SMS 201-995, octreotide) in 178 acromegalic patients: results from the international multicenter acromegaly study group. In: Lamberts SWJ, ed. *Sandostatin in the treatment of acromegaly.* Berlin: Springer-Verlag, 1988:117–25.
8. Ezzat S, Forster MJ, Berchtold P, Redelmeier D, Boerlin V, Harris AG. Acromegaly: clinical and biochemical features in 500 patients. *Medicine* 1994;73:233–40.
9. Bates AS, Van't Hoff W, Jones JM, Clayton RN. An audit of outcome of treatment in acromegaly. *Q J Med* 1993;86:293–9.
10. Wright AD, Hill DM, Lowy C, Fraser TR. Mortality in acromegaly. *Q J Med* 1970;39:1–16.
11. Melmed S. Acromegaly. *N Engl J Med* 1990;322:966–77.
12. Melmed S, Braunstein GD, Horvath E, et al. Pathophysiology of acromegaly. *Endocrine Rev* 1983;4:271–90. 1983.
13. Herman V, Fagin J, Gonsky R, Kovacs K, Melmed S. Clonal origin of pituitary adenomas. *J Clin Endocrinol Metab* 1990;61:1185–9.
14. Vallar L, Spada A, Giannattasio G. Altered Gs and adenylate cyclase activity in human GH-secreting pituitary adenomas. *Nature* 1987;330:566–8.
15. Clementi E, Malgarctti N, Meldolesi J, et al. A new constitutively activating mutation of the Gs protein alpha subunit-gsp oncogene is found in human pituitary tumours. *Oncogene* 1990;5:1059.
16. Landis CA, Masters SB, Spada A, Pace AM, Bourne HR, Valler L. GTPase inhibiting mutations activate the alpha chain of Gs, and stimulate adenylyl cyclase in human pituitary tumors. *Nature* 1989;340:692–6.
17. Melmed S, Ho K, Klibanski A, Reichlin S, Thorner M. Clinical review 75: recent advances in pathogenesis, diagnosis, and management of acromegaly. *J Clin Endocrinol Metab* 1995;80:3395–402.
18. Riedel M, Günther T, von zur Mühlen A, Brabant G. The pulsatile GH secretion in acromegaly: hypothalamic or pituitary origin? *Clin Endocrinol* 1992;37:233–9.
19. Attanasio R, Cozzi R, Oppizzi G, et al. Persistence of somatostatinergic tone in acromegaly. *Eur J Endocrinol* 1995;132:27–31.
20. Faglia G, Arosio M, Bazzoni N. Ectopic acromegaly. *Endocrinol Metab Clin North Am* 1992;21:575–95.
21. Melmed S, Rushakoff RJ. Ectopic pituitary and hypothalamic hormone syndromes. *Endocrinol Metab Clin North Am* 1987;16:805.
22. Melmed S, Ezrin C, Kovacs K, et al. Acromegaly due to secretion of growth hormone by an ectopic pancreatic islet-cell tumor. *N Engl J Med* 1985;312:9.
23. Kovacs K, Horvath E. Pathology of growth hormone producing tumors of the human pituitary. *Semin Diagn Pathol* 1986;3:18.
24. Ikuyama S, Nawata H, Kato KI, et al. Specific somatostatin receptors on human pituitary adenoma cell membranes. *J Clin Endocrinol Metab* 1985;6:666.
25. Bruns C, Weckbecker G, Raulf F, et al. Molecular pharmacology of somatostatin-receptor subtypes. *Ann NY Acad Sci* 1994;733:138–46.
26. Miller GM, Alexander JM, Bikkal HA, Katznelson L, Zervas NT, Klibanski A. Somatostatin receptor subtype gene expression in pituitary adenomas. *J Clin Endocrinol Metab* 1995;80:1386–92.
27. Greenman Y, Melmed S. Heterogenous expression of two somatostatin receptor subtypes in pituitary tumors. *J Clin Endocrinol Metab* 1994;78:398.
28. Reubi JC, Landolt AM. The growth hormone responses to octreotide in acromegaly correlate with adenoma somatostatin receptor status. *J Clin Endocrinol Metab* 1989;68:844–50.
29. Vezina JL, Maltais R. La selle turcique dans acromegalie. Etude radiologique. *Neurochirurgie* 1973(suppl 2):35.
30. Guiot G, Oproiu A, Hertzog E, Fredy D. Adenomes hypophysaires. *EMC Paris* 1969;17:340.

CHAPTER 4

Clinical Features of Acromegaly

The consequences of GH excess are typified in acromegaly. Hypersecretion of GH affects virtually all organs and tissues, causing widespread disturbances of morphology, endocrine function, and metabolism (Table 2). There is increased production of IGF-I, the anabolic actions of which lead to increased tissue growth. Muscle mass and soft-tissue mass increase, and all visceral organs are enlarged. Furthermore, GH stimulates fibroblast proliferation, which causes increased thickening of connective tissue. Soft-tissue enlargement involving the tongue and pharynx and larynx are often sufficiently severe to cause airway obstruction during sleep (sleep apnea syndrome). GH also has other actions not mediated by IGF-I, such as its anti-insulin, lipolytic, and anti-natriuretic properties. Its antagonistic effects on insulin cause glucose intolerance or diabetes mellitus in about 25% of patients. Its lipolytic action probably explains the decreased fat mass often seen in patients with acromegaly. The anti-insulin and sodium-retaining properties of GH are believed to be responsible for increased total body sodium and water and for the frequent occurrence of hypertension. This increased salt and water retention also contributes significantly to soft-tissue swelling, which is the cause of the entrapment neuropathy (carpal tunnel syndrome) frequently observed in acromegaly.

TABLE 2. *Clinical features of acromegaly*

General effects	Cardiovascular and respiratory effects
Soft tissue swelling	Hypertension
Acral enlargement	Cardiac enlargement
Musculoskeletal/neurological effects	Fatigue
Arthralgia	Tongue enlargement
Prognathism	Sleep apnea syndrome
Arthropathy	Daytime somnolence
Pareasthesia	Voice changes
Carpal tunnel syndrome	Gastrointestinal effects
Local tumor effects	Colonic polyps
Visual impairment	Enlarged organ size
Headaches	Psychosexual effects
Pituitary infarction	Decreased libido
Cranial nerve impingement	Menstrual disturbance
Cutaneous effects	Impotence
Cosmetic disfigurement	Depression/decreased vitality
Increased sweating	
Acne	
Greasy skin	
Skin tags	
Endocrine and metabolic effects	
Carbohydrate intolerance	
Diabetes mellitus	
Hyperphosphatemia/hypercalcuria	
Hyperlipidemia	
Goiter	
Hyperprolactinemia	

LOCAL MANIFESTATIONS

Growth of a pituitary adenoma beyond the confines of the sella turcica may compress local structures, producing symptoms such as headache, visual impairment, elevated intracranial pressure, and cranial nerve paralysis. In rare cases, expansion of a pituitary tumor into the adjacent cavernous sinuses may lead to vascular engorgement around the eye, causing proptosis.

Headache

This is a common local manifestation of acromegaly, occurring in up to 60% of patients (1–3). Although local pressure effects are believed to be responsible for acromegalic headaches, there are some doubts as to whether this is the only explanation. There appears to be no correlation between tumor size or suprasellar extension and the incidence of headache, and Molitch (4) has noted that headaches in patients with GH-secreting pituitary tumors tend to be more common than in patients with other pituitary adenomas of similar size. Headache responds well to all forms of treatment. Interestingly, the somatostatin analogue octreotide is highly effective in the rapid treatment of headache in acromegaly, which might be explained by a direct analgesic effect via somatostatin receptors (5).

Visual Disturbances

Both the optic chiasm and sections of the optic nerves lie above the superior surface of the pituitary gland (Figs. 25 and 26). Suprasellar expansion of a pituitary tumor can impinge on the optic chiasm and cause a visual field deficit, which is typically a bitemporal hemianopia with or without a central scotoma (Figs. 27 and 28). Although this feature, when it occurs, is quite typical of a large pituitary adenoma, visual field defects in general are present in only 4–5.2% of acromegalic patients at presentation. The visual field deficit may be either uni- or bilateral, although it often begins in one eye and progresses to involve both visual fields as the tumor expands. Many regions of the visual field can be affected, depending on the direction of tumor extension and the resulting involvement of different fibers within the optic chiasm. Visual acuity may also be lost. Other ophthalmologic manifestations of pituitary tumors include central scotoma, optic atrophy, and pupillary defects. Therefore, Goldmann perimetry, Snellen chart testing, and fundoscopy are required as a minimum for investigation of vision in acromegaly.

Cranial Nerve Involvement

The lateral walls of the sella turcica are composed of the cavernous sinuses, which contain parts of the oculomotor (III) and trochlear (IV) nerves, the ophthalmic (V1) and maxillary (V2) divisions of the trigeminal nerve, and the abducens (VI) nerve. Significant lateral expansion of a pituitary tumor into the cavernous sinus can impinge on these nerves and may produce symptoms of cranial nerve paralysis. Ophthalmoplegia, ptosis, pupillary abnormalities, trigeminal pain or parasthesia, and decreased reflexes may occur.

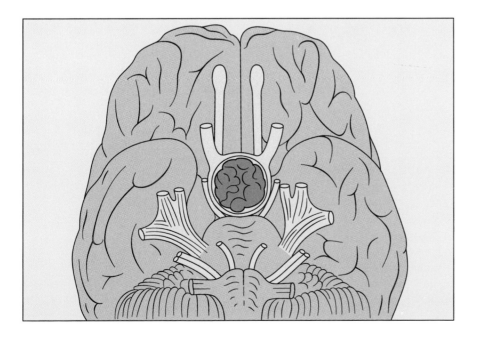

FIG. 25. Inferior view of pituitary adenoma compressing the optic chiasm.

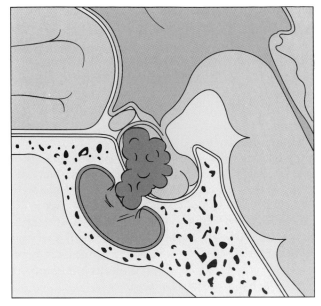

FIG. 26. Lateral section of pituitary adenoma invading the sphenoid sinus and compressing the optic chiasm.

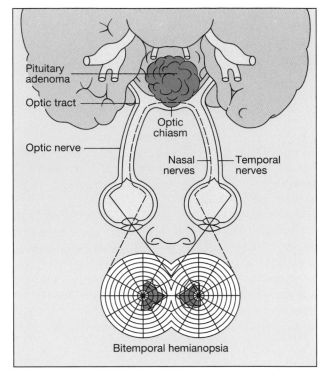

Pituitary adenoma

Optic tract

Optic nerve

Optic chiasm

Nasal nerves — Temporal nerves

Bitemporal hemianopsia

FIG. 27. Compression of the optic chiasm causing visual field defects.

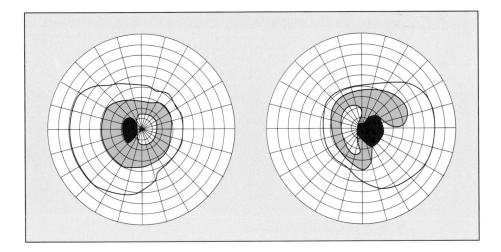

FIG. 28. Visual field defects associated with acromegaly.

Papilledema

Expansion of a pituitary adenoma superiorly may rarely lead to the obstruction of the III ventricle, leading to a buildup in cerebrospinal fluid and elevated intracranial pressure. However, because of the degree of tumor expansion required to obstruct the III ventricle, it is highly unlikely that papilledema would occur independent of more obvious local and systemic effects.

METABOLIC AND ENDOCRINE MANIFESTATIONS OF ACROMEGALY

Carbohydrate Metabolism

Growth hormone is often classified in the literature as a "diabetogenic" hormone, because it antagonizes the action of insulin and stimulates hepatic glucose mobilization (6–8). Acromegalic patients have chronically elevated GH levels and consequently 25–50% of cases suffer impairments of carbohydrate tolerance. Indeed, the failure of an oral glucose load to suppress GH secretion is one of the standard diagnostic tests in suspected acromegaly. Insulin sensitivity may be decreased (9) and insulin resistance may occur in acromegalic patients, in association with hyperinsulinemia (10). As acromegaly progresses, up to 30% of patients develop diabetes mellitus, which may be associated with lowered insulin levels, although few patients require exogenous insulin treatment. Peripheral glucose uptake and metabolism are decreased in acromegaly, which also serves to perturb normal glucose dynamics (11).

Decreasing GH secretion in acromegaly, either surgically (12), by radiation (13), or by octreotide (14) or bromocriptine (15), improves carbohydrate intolerance and can reverse overt diabetes in many cases. The negative impact of diabetes mellitus in acromegaly, although not fully evaluated, probably adds to the rate of mortality from cardiovascular disease.

Lipid Metabolism

Growth hormone is a lipolytic hormone (16,17), and patients with acromegaly consequently demonstrate elevated plasma triglyceride concentrations (18). This abnormally elevated fat mobilization may also be explained by parallel GH/IGF–I-related interference with fatty acid storage mechanisms, such as lipoprotein lipase (19) or by coexisting diabetes mellitus. The effects of acromegaly and treatment on lipoprotein levels have been recently studied. Increased levels of lipoprotein (a) and triglycerides may contribute to the increased cardiovascular morbidity and mortality associated with untreated acromegaly. Treatment

with surgery (20) or the somatostatin analogue octreotide (21) has been shown to reverse this increase. Because approximately 50% of patients with acromegaly have hypertension, the concomitant presence of hyperlipidemia may increase morbidity and mortality from cerebrovascular and cardiovascular disease.

Thyroid Function

Approximately 10% of acromegalic patients suffer from hyperthyroidism, usually caused by a nodular goiter. Such overgrowth of the thyroid is believed to occur in up to 40% of patients. It is not known whether this reflects GH/IGF–I-stimulated growth of the thyroid gland or whether it involves altered TSH secretion, which occurs in 20–35% of patients. As in the case with diabetes in acromegaly, hyperthyroidism can contribute significantly to morbidity because of its associated hypertension and disorders of body composition.

SYSTEMIC MANIFESTATIONS

Cutaneous and Soft-Tissue Manifestations

Increased GH and IGF-I levels in acromegaly lead to a number of striking skin changes (Table 3). Soft-tissue swelling and acral growth are responsible for producing the obvious changes in body habitus and facial appearance that typify acromegaly. Increases in the breadth of hands and feet may lead to ill-fitting rings, gloves, and shoes (Figs. 29 and 30). Facial soft tissue swelling can cause skin creases to become very pronounced, a condition known as *cutis verticis gyrata* (Fig. 31). Soft-tissue swelling is mainly determined by increased IGF-I concentrations (22), which

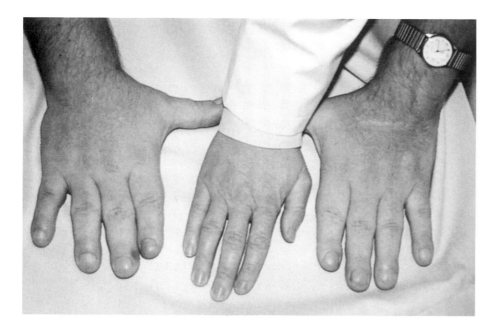

FIG. 29. Photograph showing acromegalic hands compared with a normal hand. Note the characteristic increase in breadth of the acromegalic hands. (Courtesy of A. Beckers and A. Stevenaert, University of Liege, Belgium.)

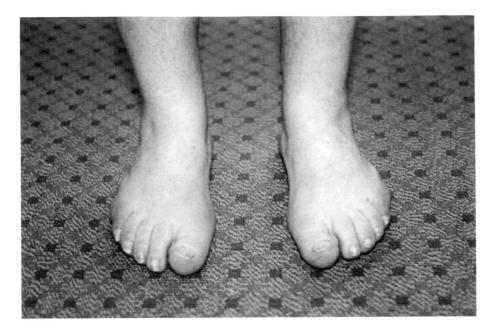

FIG. 30. The acromegalic patient requires progressively larger shoes because the feet become enlarged in breadth. (Courtesy of A. Beckers and A. Stevenaert, University of Liege, Belgium.)

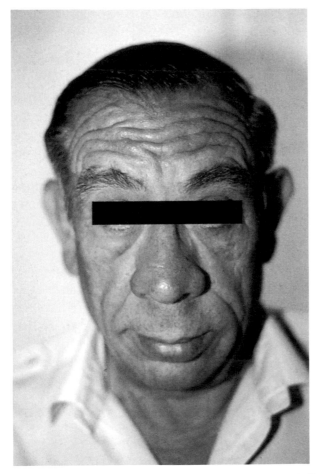

FIG. 31. Furrowing of the forehead in an acromegalic patient. (Courtesy of A. Beckers and A. Stevenaert, University of Liege, Belgium.)

TABLE 3. Cutaneous manifestations of acromegaly

Soft-tissue swelling
    Increased hand breadth (increased glove and ring size)
    Increased foot breadth (increased shoe size)
    Facial swelling
Cutis verticis gyrata
Greasy skin (seborrhea)
Increased sweating (hyperhidrosis)
Skin tags
Nail thickening
Acanthosis nigricans (velvety hyperpigmentation)

leads to increased amounts of glycosaminoglycans in the dermis (23), causing edema. Sodium and water retention typical to acromegaly, compound this edema. Increased collagen synthesis and bony changes also cause deformation of facial features (see Musculoskeletal and Neurological Manifestations). Soft-tissue swelling responds very well to therapy, often improving significantly within weeks of treatment (medical, surgical, or radiation). Patients commonly suffer from increased perspiration (hyperhidrosis) and greasy skin (seborrhea), which is due to overactivity of sweat and sebaceous glands, respectively. This leads to an offensive body odor, which requires increased use of expensive cosmetics and antiperspirants. Furthermore, some individuals with acromegaly suffer form acne vulgaris, which is probably caused by sebaceous gland overactivity. Again, effective treatment of acromegaly improves these symptoms, which obviously has a major effect on patients' self-image.

Musculoskeletal and Neurologic Manifestations

GH and IGF-I are major determinants of skeletal growth and muscle bulk, whereas the effect of GH/IGF-I on nerve growth and physiology is less clear. Patients with acromegaly commonly report symptoms related to bony and cartilaginous changes, and the generalized fatigue often experienced may be related to neuromuscular pathology.

Arthropathy and Bone Malformations

Pituitary gigantism is caused by abnormal longitudinal bone growth in response to GH hypersecretion in prepubescent patients, who have open, active epiphyseal plates. The majority of pituitary tumors occur in adults, who suffer from arthropathies, mandibular enlargement, and disfiguring bony overgrowth of other areas of the skull.

Arthralgia is one of the most common complaints of acromegalic patients, with a rate of approximately 75% reported in major rheumatologic studies (24,25). The pain is caused by the stimulatory effects of GH (26) and IGF-1 (27) on bone and cartilaginous tissue within joints. In osteoblasts and chondrocytes, local IGF-1 activity appears to be regulated by GH (28,29). Moreover, locally produced IGFBPs may be important in the regulation of bone growth (30). Therefore, chronically elevated GH in acromegaly leads to increased local IGF-I production within the joints and articular tissues. Collagenous overgrowth occurs, followed by misalignment and destabilization of joint architecture. Subsequently, joint spaces widen and osteoarthritis occurs as the affected joints gradually become damaged, laying down new cartilage which eventually calcifies. Furthermore, it has been suggested that GH and IGF-I also stimulate collagen production within tendon, causing laxity and leading to further joint destabilization (31). As noted above, GH/IGF-I work together to stimulate osteoblast activity, and this leads to bony degenerative change in areas adjacent to joints, producing a radiologic picture similar to that of nonacromegalic osteoarthritis. On x-ray, calcification of tendinous and ligamentous insertions (enthesopathy), widening of joint spaces, and tufting of distal phalanges may be observed. A complete list of radiologic findings in acromegaly is shown in Table 4. Podgorski and colleagues (24) have reported spinal and peripheral abnormalities in 47% and 74% of acromegalic patients, respectively. Hip, shoulder, knee, hand, and ribcage joints were commonly affected in this study.

The development of a prominent mandible (prognathism), with malocclusion of the teeth, may be noted by acromegalic patients themselves or by their dentists. This feature is illustrated in Fig. 32. In addition, as the dimensions of the mouth alter with the progressive growth of the lower jaw in response to high GH and IGF-I levels (see above), chronic ill-fitting of dentures may be noted. Patients with acromegaly may suffer temporomandibular

TABLE 4. Radiologic findings in acromegalic joint disease
Increased joint space diameter
Decreased joint space diameter (severe disease)
Tufting of distal phalanges
Enthesopathy
Angular joint deformities
Osteophyte formation
Articular surface calcification
Eburnation
Subchondral cyst formation
Costochondral joint calcification and enlargement
Vertebral body enlargement

joint dysfunction, a painful syndrome caused by malocclusion and neuromuscular factors (32).

Bony malformations of the skull add to the general disfiguring effects of soft-tissue swelling in acromegaly. Although treatment may improve soft tissue changes, long-term skeletal changes may require maxillofacial corrective surgery. Little has been published about corrective surgery in acromegaly, but excellent results have been achieved (33,34). After successful treatment, the possibility of such reconstructive surgery should be raised with patients when appropriate.

Neurologic and Muscular Effects

Fatigue is commonly reported by patients with active acromegaly, and GH/IGF–I-related changes in muscle mass and neuromuscular function may be the cause of this symptom. In keeping with the general increase in organ size, acromegaly is associated with muscle fiber hypertrophy, although differential patterns of muscle fiber enlargement and shrinkage can be found (35–37). Despite increased muscle mass, patients experience weakness and electromyographic (EMG) alterations that are consistent with a proximal myopathy (38,39). Treatment of acromegaly is associated with an improvement in patient well-being and vitality, although the precise impact of therapy on muscle changes per se has yet to be assessed.

The peripheral nerves themselves are abnormal in acromegaly. Jamal et al. (40) reported that reflexes, temperature, light touch, superficial pain, and vibration sensations were decreased in patients with acromegaly, often asymptomatically. Ulnar or popliteal nerves were found to be enlarged in approximately 42% of patients, and neurophysiologic measures were significantly depressed in 12 of 14 criteria assessed compared with healthy subjects. These authors and others (41) found no relationship to GH levels or carbohydrate intolerance (i.e., coexisting diabetes mellitus). Dinn and Dinn (42) performed a pathologic analysis of peripheral nerve biopsy specimens from acromegalic patients and reported mild to severe random seg-

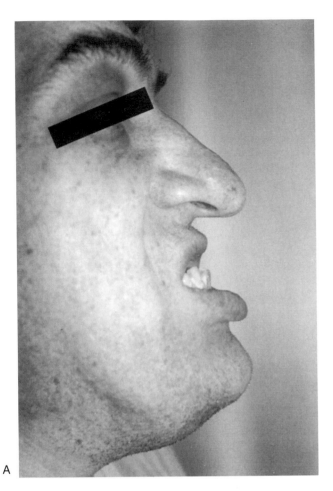

A

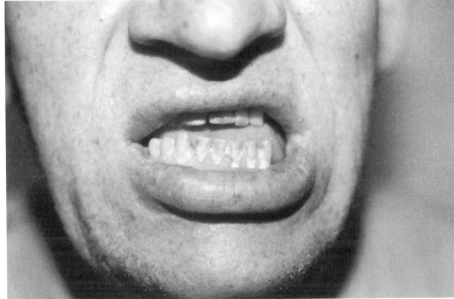

B

FIG. 32. Signs of acromegaly that may be noted by the dentist. **A:** Prognathism. Protrusion of the low mandible is marked in this patient and malocclusion of the teeth can be seen. **B:** Increased interdental spaces due to widening of the mandible. (Courtesy of A. Beckers and A. Stevenaert, University of Liege, Belgium.)

mental demyelination of small diameter nerve fibers. The authors noted that end-stage neuropathic changes appeared to involve irreversible "onion bulb" Schwann cell deformities.

Paresthesias of the extremities are reported in about 50% of acromegaly cases (43), with carpal tunnel syndrome a presenting complaint in 6% of cases (44). Carpal tunnel syndrome is probably caused primarily by the increase in extracellular fluid volume, which causes compression of nerves in the wrist. However, paresthesia may be exacerbated by pathological changes to the nerve itself, as noted above. In their review, Lieberman and Hoffman reported that carpal tunnel syndrome resolves following treatment, but may take 6 weeks to 2 years to become apparent (45).

Cardiovascular Manifestations

Hypertension

Hypertension has been reported in 25–50% of patients with acromegaly and is a major contributor to mortality from cardiovascular disease. Although the precise mechanism of acromegalic hypertension remains unknown, it appears that sodium and water retention is a major determining factor. GH has a direct effect on renal sodium pump activity (46), and this may provide the explanation for both hypertension and increased extracellular water volume in acromegaly (47). Other groups have reported a possible link between plasma insulin levels and hypertension in acromegaly (48,49). Ezzat et al. (43) noted in their series of 500 patients that older patients had higher systolic and diastolic blood pressure than younger patients, but there was no correlation between GH levels and blood pressure. Therefore, the severity of hypertension in acromegaly may be a function of the duration of abnormally increased GH levels. This would be in line with the negative impact of chronically raised GH on life expectancy, as noted by Rajasoorya and colleagues (50).

Cardiac Manifestations

Excessive levels of GH and IGF-I have a significant effect on cardiac morphology and function (Table 5) (51). Concentric cardiomegaly, caused by myocardial hypertrophy and increased connective tissue synthesis, is the most common cardiac abnormality seen in acromegaly (52). Although much of this enlargement reflects overall visceromegaly, Saccà and co-workers have pointed out that echocardiographic (53,54) and autopsy studies (55) demonstrate that heart size is greater than would be expected from body weight. As with other acromegalic complications, it may be that the duration of GH hypersecretion is of greater significance in the progression of cardiac disease in acromegaly than the peak GH levels. Cardiomegaly is exacerbated by hypertension, which is probably due to

TABLE 5. *Cardiac manifestations of acromegaly*
Ventricular hypertrophy
Valvular lesions
Interstitial fibrosis
Collagen overgrowth
Mononuclear leukocyte infiltration
Myocarditis
Arrhythmias
Impaired diastolic filling
Impaired exercise performance

expansion of the extracellular fluid volume. It is important to note that asymptomatic patients also have demonstrable cardiac abnormalities (56), which makes early diagnosis and treatment a necessity.

Patients with acromegaly demonstrate arrhythmias, which are predominantly ventricular (57) and worsen with disease duration (58). Saccà et al. (52) have suggested that interstitial fibrosis is the precipitating factor in ventricular arrhythmias.

Cardiac performance at rest and during exercise is affected in acromegaly. Patients exhibit disorders of diastolic filling at rest, whereas systolic function may be normal. Fazio et al. (59) have noted that during exercise, acromegalic patients do not experience a rise in systolic ejection fraction, a highly abnormal finding that impairs exercise tolerance significantly. As disease progresses, cardiac symptoms can worsen and lead to heart failure, which represents a major threat to life. Cardiac disease in acromegaly is complicated by the common occurrence of hypertension, which decreases ventricular diastolic function (60). Surgical and medical treatment of acromegaly have been shown to improve cardiac performance significantly (61–66) and even to reverse myocardial pathology, such as intracellular myofibrillolysis (67).

It has been argued that certain phenomena seen in the diseased acromegalic heart, such as lymphocyte infiltration and interstitial fibrosis, indicate the existence of a specific acromegalic cardiomyopathy. In their comprehensive review, Saccà and colleagues (52) point out that these pathologic features appear to be directly attributable to GH/IGF-I excess, and that treatment which reduces GH/IGF-I levels (i.e., a somatostatin analogue such as octreotide) can reverse cardiopathic changes. Other parallel pathologic conditions, such as diabetes mellitus and hypertension, can cause significant heart disease in their own right. However, patients with uncomplicated acromegaly (i.e., without diabetes or hypertension) have impaired functioning of both ventricles in diastole and systole. In conclusion, it is likely that heart disease in acromegaly is caused by a combination of a specific GH/IGF–I-related cardiopathy and the more well-known negative effects of hypertension, hyperlipidemia, respiratory disease, and diabetes mellitus on the heart.

Vascular Complications

The precise incidence of coronary artery and cerebrovascular disease in acromegaly is a controversial subject, and many conflicting data have been published. In their review, Saccà et al. (52) stated that coronary artery disease rates of 3–37% have been reported in various studies, although it appears from perfusion studies that the rate is nearer 20–37%. However, the mortality from cerebrovascular and coronary artery disease in acromegaly is high, at 3.3- and 3-fold the rates in the general population, respectively. The separate and combined impact of hypertension, diabetes mellitus, and hyperlipidemia on atheroma formation in acromegaly remains to be assessed. The importance of cardiovascular disease as a cause of mortality in acromegalic patients (40–60%) necessitates prompt and effective treatment to improve life expectancy.

Cancer

Epidemiologic evidence has shown that acromegaly is associated with increased morbidity and mortality. As noted previously, the major determinants of mortality are vascular disease and respiratory illness. Although in early epidemiologic studies the rate of cancer-related deaths was not increased (68–70), studies since then have demonstrated an increased incidence of malignant disease in acromegaly (71,72). Many types of cancer have been reported in acromegalic patients, e.g., colorectal, breast, renal, thyroid, and hematologic malignancies. Alexander et al. (73) reported that cancer in general accounted for approximately 15% of all deaths in acromegaly. Later work by Nabarro (1) demonstrated a greatly increased incidence of cancer in female patients only, who had four times the expected rate of breast cancer. Barzilay and colleagues (74) observed that acromegalic patients were almost 2.5 times more likely to develop malignant tumors than control subjects (patients with endocrine-inactive pituitary tumors). The largest patient population studied this far (albeit retrospectively) was reported by Ron et al. (75), who studied 1,041 men with acromegaly discharged form the Veterans Administration hospitals between 1969 and 1985. These authors observed an increased incidence of gastrointestinal cancers, such as those of the colon, stomach, and esophagus (standard incidence ratio 2.0), with colon cancer being the main determinant of this result.

Although malignancy in general appears to be increased in acromegaly, the published literature provides persuasive evidence only in the case of colon cancer. Colonic polyps, which are the benign early stage of colon cancer, are more common in acromegalic patients, compared with the general population. Ezzat et al. (76) reported that of 8 of 23 (35%) acromegalic patients had colonic polyps, and Terzolo et al. (77) found hyperplastic polyps in 12 of 31 patients (38%) in a recent study. Klein et al. (78) reported a prevalence of colonic polyps as high as 53%. Interestingly, Leav-

itt and colleagues (79) have noted that multiple skin tags may be a reliable and noninvasive cutaneous marker for colonic polyps in the general population. On the basis of these and other reports (80–84), Ezzat and Melmed (85) concluded in their review that in patients aged 50 or over, a history of colonic polyps or multiple skin tags appears to be a positive predictor of neoplasia in acromegaly. This was underscored by the recent work of Delhougne and colleagues (86), who reported a prevalence of hyperplastic polyps of 24.3% (compared with 4.4% in control subjects) in a study of 103 acromegalic patients. Therefore, acromegalic patients in the at-risk group should be closely managed by a gastroenterologist, and regular colonoscopies every 1 to 2 years are probably warranted.

In the case of other malignancies, little strong evidence exists. It must be borne in mind that GH has been shown to promote cancer growth in tissue culture and animal studies, such as the pioneering work of Moon et al. (87). In addition, IGF-I may work at a cellular and genomic level to promote oncogenesis. Therefore, until more long-term experience with acromegaly and the beneficial effects of medical and surgical treatment provide us with definitive evidence, doctors should be constantly aware of the possibility of cancer, colorectal and otherwise, in acromegalic patients under their care.

Renal Effects and Electrolye Balance

Calcium, phosphate, sodium, and water homeostasis are affected in acromegaly (88–90). The levels of calcium and phosphate ions are regulated by the kidney (excretion/ retention), the gut (absorption), and the actions of vitamin D and parathyroid hormone. As was outlined above, bone turnover is stimulated by GH/IGF-I, thus promoting hypercalcemia and hyperphosphatemia. Added to this is the observation that vitamin D activity is enhanced in acromegaly, thus leading to increased gut absorption of calcium (91). In parallel with this, phosphate absorption in the kidney is stimulated in acromegaly (92). It is not known whether parathyroid hormone levels are increased or decreased in acromegaly, as conflicting evidence has been published (93,94). Treatment of acromegaly with the somatostatin analogue octreotide causes an increase in parathyroid hormone levels (95), whereas surgical adenomectomy does not affect it (96). In cases where acromegaly coexists with primary hyperparathyroidism, multiple endocrine neoplasia type I (MEN I) must be suspected strongly, and thoroughly investigated. With these abnormalities in calcium and phosphate regulation, the risk of renal stones should be recognized. Pines and Olchovsky found evidence of urolithiasis in eight of 64 acromegalic patients, studied retrospectively (97). They noted that hypercalciuria was present in 42–68% of cases of acromegaly in a review of published literature, while renal stones were reported in 6–7% of acromegalic patients. In Pines and Olchovsky's series, three patients had their renal stones noted before acromegaly was diagnosed. This further underlines the fact that all clinical specialists should be aware of acromegaly as a rare cause of commonly presenting complaints.

Sodium and water retention occurs in acromegaly, and may be an important factor in causing hypertension. This may be mediated at the level of the renal tubules, via stimulation of sodium transport (98), or via an effect on the renin–angiotensin system, or aldosterone (99). This important aspect of the pathophysiology of acromegaly is complex and only partially understood. Increased body water and sodium levels are also an important cause of soft tissue swelling and compression neuropathies, such as carpal tunnel syndrome.

Body Composition and Energy Metabolism

GH and IGF-I have significant effects on body water and energy stores, and specific alterations in body composition and energy metabolism are observed in acromegaly (100,101). As stated above, lipolysis is increased in acromegaly, and this leads to decreased body fat deposits compared with those of nonacromegalic individuals. Body water (extracellular fluid, plasma volume) is increased in acromegaly, probably because of sodium retention by the kidney, and this leads to much of the disfiguring soft-tissue swelling that is a hallmark of active acromegaly (102). Furthermore, this increase in body water is the most likely cause of carpal tunnel syndrome, which is seen to some degree in approximately 30% of patients with acromegaly. Successful treatment of acromegaly (transsphenoidal hypophysectomy, radiotherapy, or medical therapy) is associated with a decrease in fluid retention, body weight, and lean body mass (103–105), which is probably the reason for improvements in soft-tissue swelling and nerve entrapment after treatment. However, these effects are seen at post-treatment GH levels <5 μg/L but are less pronounced at higher concentrations.

Whole-body energy metabolism and substrate oxidation in acromegaly were studied recently by O'Sullivan and colleagues (106). Interestingly, they found that carbohydrate and lipid oxidation were increased and decreased, respectively, which is the opposite of what was expected from short-term GH administration studies. In addition, impaired insulin response and IGF-I levels appeared to play an important role in the regulation of energy expenditure and substrate oxidation.

Sleep Apnea Syndrome

A patent upper airway must be maintained during sleep to provide adequate oxygenation and alveolar gas exchange. Central respiratory drive and a stable and coordinated system of upper airway muscles and soft tissue are necessary to prevent hypopnea and apnea. Sleep apnea syndrome, which is characterized by repeated hypopnic and apneic attacks during sleep, may be caused either by disturbed central drive or by structural collapse of the pharynx.

Grunstein et al. (107) reported that sleep-related upper airway obstruction is experienced by over 50% of patients with acromegaly. Undoubtedly, enlargement of the tongue and pharyngeal structures contributes to the development of obstructive sleep apnea (Fig. 33), but central apnea has also been reported in a large proportion of acromegalic patients. Those patients with central apnea have higher GH and IGF-I levels than acromegalic patients with obstructive-type sleep apnea. This may be due to in part to a higher ventilatory response to increased CO_2, which may be an indicator of decreased chemoreceptor drive (108). Although the exact role of excess GH/IGF-I in central apnea is unknown, it should be noted that central and obstructive forms of apnea coexist in many cases and that improved stability of the upper airway may subsequently decrease the frequency of central apnea (109,110).

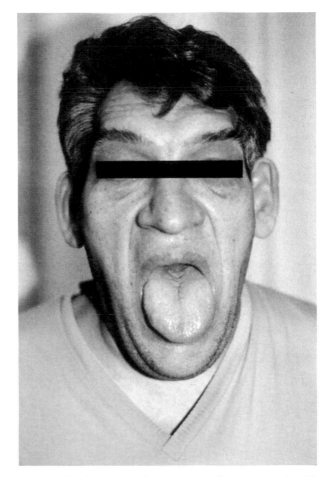

FIG. 33. Further typical features of acromegaly. The acromegalic facies is characterized by prognathism, coarse features, and prominent supra- and suborbital ridges. The nasal and the auricular cartilage are thickened and the tongue enlarged. (Courtesy of A. Beckers and A. Stevenaert, University of Liege, Belgium.)

Far from being a benign condition, sleep apnea syndrome has significant effects on patients' well-being. Daytime somnolence, fatigue, irritability, and poor concentration have a negative impact on the patient's ability to work and interact socially. Acromegalic patients with sleep apnea syndrome have decreased durations of REM sleep (111). In addition, sleep apnea syndrome is associated with inappropriate blood oxygen and CO_2 levels which can have seriously deleterious effects on the heart over the long term. This latter point is significant when the already compromised state of cardiac function due to direct effects of GH/IGF-I on heart size is considered.

Treatment of acromegaly, either surgically or medically, has been reported to improve sleep apnea syndrome. Astrom et al. (112) reported that daytime sleepiness and decreased REM sleep duration improved in nine young acromegalic patients, although Pelttari et al. (113) have recently noted that sleep disturbances, although improved, may still exist after successful surgery. After 6 months of treatment with octreotide (100–500 μg t.i.d. s.c.), Grunstein

et al. (109) reported that 19 patients with acromegaly and sleep apnea had significantly decreased respiratory disturbance and total apnea time. Interestingly, there was no correlation between the nocturnal breathing improvements and decreases in GH and IGF-I levels. It may be that octreotide achieves at least some of its beneficial effects by increasing REM sleep duration, while increasing the diameter of the upper airway (Figs. 34 and 35).

Psychological Aspects of Acromegaly

Because the physical manifestations of acromegaly are so profound and have such a negative impact on patients' physical health, the effect of this disease on the individual's mental state has been relatively ignored. It is well known that patients with acromegaly suffer greatly from depression and fatigue. However, it is not yet clear if this is due to the debilitating and deforming effects of the disease or can be explained by a direct effect of GH/IGF-I. Few standardized psychometric trials have been performed in acro-

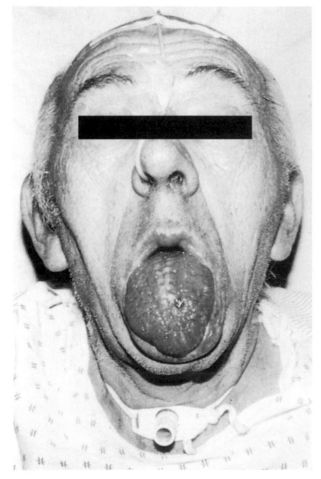

FIG. 34. Acromegaly in a patient suffering from obstructive sleep apnea before octreotide. Note the massively enlarged tongue, tracheotomy for airway obstruction and intranasal feeding tube.

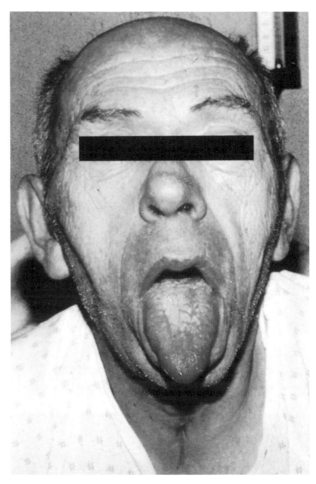

FIG. 35. Same patient after 6 months of treatment with octreotide. The size of the tongue was reduced by half. Tracheotomy and nasal tube have been removed. The patient no longer suffers from sleep apnea. (Courtesy of S. Reichlin, Tufts University, Boston, MA.)

megaly, although the possibility of psychiatric illness in pituitary disease has been recognized for many years (114), and treatment approaches were suggested by Bleuler in the 1950s (115). Abed et al. (116) found no increased rate of psychiatric disease in acromegaly, whereas an anxiety and personality-based study by Sablowski and colleagues (117) and other work (118) have shown acromegalic patients to have specific ambition and motivational losses. Ezzat (119) published the results of a survey of psychological changes in 39 patients with acromegaly. Self-image was worsened among one-third of female patients (two-thirds of unmarried female patients), and marked withdrawal in interpersonal relationships was noted in 42% and 56% of female and male patients, respectively.

In summary, it is common for patients with acromegaly to suffer from depression and poor self-image. This psychopathology is undoubtedly related to the physical changes and endocrinologic disturbances associated with acromegaly. Therefore, it should be expected that improved well-being after treatment will be followed by amelioration of mood disorders. Large-scale, well-designed prospective psychometric studies are required to define the beneficial effect of treatment on the mental state of acromegalic patients.

Sexual Dysfunction

Loss of libido occurs in over half of patients with acromegaly and is associated with a large amount of personal stress for both the patient and his or her partner. Molitch (120) has noted that decreased libido or impotence was the presenting symptom in 3% of cases of acromegaly. This should underscore the need for all health care workers to be aware of the multiple manifestations of acromegaly. Although no specific work has studied the effects of treatment on loss of libido, patients appear to improve in parallel with overall symptomatic amelioration. Hyperprolactinemia, which occurs in up to 30% of cases of acromegaly, appears to be a major factor in acromegaly-related sexual dysfunction in both men and women. For female acromegalic patients, amenorrhea is a major problem, afflicting over 50%. In summary, these complaints mean that acromegaly can have a serious impact on fertility and, by extension, on interpersonal relationships. The precise cause of sexual dysfunction should be ascertained, as many other factors unrelated to prolactin can interfere with normal sexual function and fertility (e.g., hypopituitarism and poor self-image), and hyperprolactinemia may be merely a complicating factor. A very sensitive specialist approach is required to deal with this complicated and highly emotion-laden problem.

REFERENCES

1. Nabarro JDN. Acromegaly. *Clin Endocrinol* 1987;26:481–512.
2. Harris AG, Prestele H, Herold K, Boerlin V. Long-term efficacy of Sandostatin (SMS 201-995, octreotide) in 178 acromegalic patients: results from the international multicenter acromegaly study group. In: Lamberts SWJ, ed. *Sandostatin in the treatment of acromegaly.* Berlin: Springer-Verlag, 1988:117–25.
3. Ezzat S, Forster MJ, Berchtold P, Redelmeier D, Boerlin V, Harris AG. Acromegaly: clinical and biochemical features in 500 patients. *Medicine* 1994;73:233–40.
4. Molitch M. Clinical manifestations of acromegaly. *Endocrinol Metab Clin North Am* 1992;21:597–614.
5. Williams G, Ball J, Lawson R, et al. Analgesic effect of somatostatin analogue (octreotide) in headache associated with pituitary tumors. *BMJ* 1987;295:247.
6. Davidson MB. Effect of growth hormone on carbohydrate and lipid metabolism. *Endocrine Rev* 1987;8:115–31.
7. Brautsch-Marrain PR, Smith D, DeFronzo RA. The effect of growth hormone on glucose metabolism and insulin secretion in man. *J Clin Endocrinol Metab* 1982;55:973–82.
8. Rizza RA, Mandarino LJ, Gerich JE. Effects of growth hormone on insulin action in man. Mechanisms of insulin resistance, impaired suppression of glucose production, and impaired stimulation of glucose utilization. *Diabetes* 1982;31:663–9.
9. Jap TS, Ho LT. Insulin secretion and sensitivity in acromegaly. *Clin Physiol Biochem* 1990;8:64–9.
10. Hansen I, Tsalikian E. Beaufrere B, Gerich J, Haymond M, Rizza R. Insulin resistance in acromegaly: defects in both hepatic and extrahepatic insulin action. *Am J Physiol* 1986;250:269–73.
11. Foss MC, Saad MJA, Paccola MGF, Paula FJA, Piccinato CE, Moreira AC. Peripheral glucose metabolism in acromegaly. *J Clin Endocrinol Metab* 1991;72:1048–53.
12. Sonksen P, Greenwood F, Ellis J, Lowy C, Rutherford A, Nabarro J. Changes of carbohydrate tolerance in acromegaly with progress of the disease and response to treatment. *J Clin Endocrinol Metab* 1967;27:1418–30.
13. Eastman RC, Gorden P, Roth J. Conventional supervoltage irradiation is an effective treatment for acromegaly. *J Clin Endocrinol Metab* 1979;48:931–40.
14. Ho KKY, Jenkins AB, Furler SM, Borkman M, Chisholm DJ. Impact of octreotide, a long-acting somatostatin analogue, on glucose tolerance and insulin sensitivity in acromegaly. *Clin Endocrinol* 1992;36:271–9.
15. Feek CM, Bevan JS, Taylor S, Brown NS, Baird JD. The effect of bromocriptine on insulin secretion and glucose tolerance in patients with acromegaly. *Clin Endocrinol* 1981;15:473–8.
16. Goodman HM, Schwartz Y, Tai LR, et al. Actions of growth hormone on adipose tissue: possible involvement of autocrine and paracrine factors. *Acta Paediatr Scand* 1990;367:132.
17. Van Vliet G, Bosson D, Craen M, et al. Comparative study of the lipolytic potencies of pituitary-derived and biosynthetic human growth hormone in hypopituitary children. *J Clin Endocrinol Metab* 1987;65:876.
18. Nikkila EA, Pelkonen R. Serum lipids in acromegaly. *Metabolism* 1975;24:829–38.
19. Murase T, Yamada N, Ohsawa N, Kosaka K, Morita S, Yoshida S. Decline of postheparin plasma lipoprotein lipase in acromegalic patients. *Metabolism* 1980;29:666–72.
20. Oscarsson J, Wiklund O, Jakobsson KE, Petruson B, Bengtsson BÅ. Serum lipoproteins in acromegaly before and 6–15 months after transsphenoidal adenomectomy. *Clin Endocrinol* 1994;41:603–8.
21. Cohen R, Chanson P, Bruckert E, et al. Effects of octreotide on lipid metabolism in acromegaly. *Horm Metab Res* 1992;24:397–400.
22. Jadresic A, Banks LM, Child DF, et al. The acromegaly syndrome. Relation between clinical features, growth hormone values and radiological characteristics of pituitary tumors. *Q J Med* 1982;51:189.
23. Matsuoka LY, Wortsman J, Kupchella CE, et al. Histochemical characterization of the cutaneous involvement of acromegaly. *Arch Intern Med* 1974;81:11.
24. Podgorski M, Robinson B, Weissberger A, Steil J, Wang S, Brooks PM. Articular manifestations of acromegaly. *Aust NZ J Med* 1988;18:28–35.
25. Dons RF, Rosselet P, Pastakia B, Doppman J, Gorden P. Arthropathy in acromegalic patients before and after treatment: a long-term follow-up study. *Clin Endocrinol* 1988;28:515–24.
26. Isaksso OG, Lindahl A, Nilsson A, et al. Mechanism of the stimulatory effect of growth hormone on longitudinal bone growth. *Endocrine Rev* 1987;8:46.

27. Trippel SB, Corvol MT, Dumontier MF, et al. Effect of somatomedin-C/insulin-like growth factor I and growth hormone on cultured growth plate and articular chondrocytes. *Pediatr Res* 1989;25:76.

28. Stracke H, Schulz A, Moeller D, et al. Effect of growth hormone on osteoblasts and demonstration of somatomedin C/IGF-I in bone organ culture. *Acta Endocrinol* 1984;107:16.

29. Nilsson A, Isgaard J, Lindahl A, et al. Regulation by growth hormone of the number of chondrocytes containing IGF-I in rat growth plate. *Science* 1986;233:571.

30. Ernst M, Rodan GA. Increased activity of insulin-like growth factor (IGF) in osteoblastic cells in the presence of growth hormone (GH): positive correlation with the presence of the GH-induced IGF-binding protein-3. *Endocrinology* 1990;127:807.

31. Liebermann SA, Björkengren AG, Hoffman AR. Rheumatologic and skeletal changes in acromegaly. *Endocrine Metab Clin North Am* 1992;21:615–31.

32. Hampton RE. Acromegaly and resulting myofascial pain and temporomandibular joint dysfunction: review of the literature and report of case. *J Am Dent Assoc* 1987;114:625–30.

33. Sugar A. Surgical correction of residual facial deformity following treatment of acromegaly. *J Max Fac Surg* 1986;14:14–7.

34. Brennan MD, Jackson IT, Keller EE, et al. Multidisciplinary management of acromegaly and its deformities. *JAMA* 1985;253:682–3.

35. Mastaglia FL. Pathological changes in skeletal muscle in acromegaly. *Acta Neuropathol* 1973;24:273–86.

36. Mastaglia FL, Barwick DD, Hall R. Myopathy in acromegaly. *Lancet* 1970;2:907–9.

37. Nagulesparen M, Trickey R, Davies MJ, et al. Muscle changes in acromegaly. *BMJ* 1976;2:914.

38. Khaleeli AA, Levy RD, Edwards RHT, et al. The neuromuscular features of acromegaly: a clinical and pathological study. *J Neurol Neurosurg Psychiatry* 1984;47:1009–15.

39. Pickett JBE, Layzer RB, Levin SR, et al. Neuromuscular complications of acromegaly. *Neurology* 1975;25:638.

40. Jamal GA, Kerr DJ, McLellan AR, Weir AI, Davies DL. Generalised peripheral nerve dysfunction in acromegaly: a study by conventional and novel neurophysiological techniques. *J Neurol Neurosurg Psychiatry* 1987;50:886–94.

41. Low PA, McLeod JG, Turtle JR, Donnelly P, Wright RG. Peripheral neuropathy in acromegaly. *Brain* 1974;97:139–52.

42. Dinn JF, Dinn EI. Natural history of peripheral neuropathy. *Q J Med* 1985;57:833–42.

43. Ezzat S, Forster MJ, Berchtold P, Redelmeier D, Boerlin V, Harris AG. Acromegaly: clinical and biochemical features in 500 patients. *Medicine* 1994;73:233–40.

44. Molitch ME. Clinical manifestations of acromegaly. *Endocrine Metab Clin North Am* 1992;21:597–614.

45. Lieberman SA, Hoffman AR. Sequelae to acromegaly: reversibility with treatment of the primary disease. *Horm Metab Res* 1990;22:313–8.

46. Shimomura Y, Lee M, Oku J, Bray GA, Glick Z. Sodium potassium dependent ATPase in hypophysectomized rats: response to growth hormone, triiodothyronine, and cortisone. *Metabolism* 1982;31:213–6.

47. Landin K, Petruson B, Jakobsson KE, Bengtsson BA. Skeletal muscle sodium and potassium changes after successful surgery in acromegaly: relation to body composition, blood glucose, plasma insulin and blood pressure. *Acta Endocrinol* 1993;128:418–22.

48. Ikeda T, Terasawa H, Ishimura M, et al. Correlation between blood pressure and plasma insulin in acromegaly. *J Intern Med* 1993;234:61–3.

49. Slowinska-Srzednicka J, Zgliczynski S, Soszynski P, Zglicznski W, Jeske W. High blood pressure and hyperinsulinaemia in acromegaly and obesity. *Clin Exp Hypertens Theory Pract* 1989;11:407–25.

50. Rajasoorya C, Holdaway IM, Wrightson P, Scott DJ, Ibbertson HK. Determinants of clinical outcome and survival in acromegaly. *Clin Endocrinol* 1994;41:95–102.

51. McGuffin WL, Sherman BM, Roth J, et al. Acromegaly and cardiovascular disorders: a prospective study. *Ann Intern Med* 1974;81:11–8.

52. Saccà L, Cittadini A, Fazio S. Growth hormone and the heart. *Endocrine Rev* 1994;15:555–73.

53. Hradec J, Marek J, Kral J, Janota T, Poloniecki J, Malik M. Long-term echocardiographic follow-up of acromegalic heart disease. *Am J Cardiol* 1993;72:205–10.

54. Fazio S, Cittadini A, Sabatini D, et al. Evidence for biventricular involvement in acromegaly: a Doppler echocardiographic study. *Eur Heart J* 1993;14:26–33.

55. Lie JT, Grossman SJ. Pathology of the heart in acromegaly: anatomic findings in 27 autopsied patients. *Am Heart J* 1980;100:41–52.

56. Morvan D, Komajda M, Grimaldi A, Turpit G, Grosgogeat Y. Cardiac hypertrophy and function in asymptomatic acromegaly. *Eur Heart J* 1991;12:666–72.

57. Kahaly G, Olshausen KV, Mohr-Kahaly S, et al. Arrhythmia profile in acromegaly. *Eur Heart J* 1992;13:51–6.

58. Kahay G, Stover C, Beyer J, Mohr-Kahaly S. Relation of endocrine and cardiac findings in acromegalics. *J Endocrinol Invest* 1992;15:13–8.

59. Fazio S, Cittadini A, Cuocolo A, et al. Impaired cardiac performance is a distinct feature of uncomplicated acromegaly. *J Clin Endocrinol Metab* 1994;79:441–6.

60. Rodrigues EA, Caruna MP, Lahiri A, Nabarro JDN, Jacobs HS, Raftery EB. Subclinical cardiac dysfunction in acromegaly: evidence for a specific disease of heart muscle. *Br Heart J* 1989;62:185–94.

61. Hayward RP, Emanuel RW, Nabarro JDN. Acromegalic heart disease: influence of treatment of acromegaly on the heart. *Q J Med* 1987;62:41–58.

62. Theusen L, Christensen SE, Weeke J, Orskov H, Henningsen P. The cardiovascular effects of octreotide treatment in acromegaly: an echocardiographic study. *Clin Endocrinol* 1989;30:619–28.

63. Merola B, Cittadini A, Colao A, et al. Chronic treatment with the somatostatin analog octreotide improves cardiac abnormalities in acromegaly. *J Clin Endocrinol Metab* 1993;77:790–3.

64. Lim MJ, Barkan AL, Buda AJ. Rapid reduction of left ventricular hypertrophy in acromegaly after suppression of growth hormone hypersecretion. *Ann Intern Med* 1992;117:719–26.

65. Chanson P, Timsit J, Masquet C, et al. Cardiovascular effects of the somatostatin analog octreotide in acromegaly. *Ann Intern Med* 1990;113:921–5.

66. Chanson P, Timsit S, Masquet C, et al. Heart failure responsive to octreotide in a patient with acromegaly. *Lancet* 1989;1:1263–4.

67. Legrand V, Beckers A, Pham VT, Demoulin JC, Stevenaert A. Dramatic improvement of severe dilated cardiomyopathy in an acromegalic patient after treatment with octreotide and trans-sphenoidal surgery. *Eur Heart J* 1994;15:1286–9.

68. Wright AD, Hill DM, Lowy C, Fraser TR. Mortality in acromegaly. *Q J Med* 1970;39:1–16.

69. Mustacchi P, Simkin MB. Occurrence of cancer in acromegaly and hypopituitarism. *Cancer* 1957;10:100–4.

70. Evans HM, Briggs JH, Dixon JS. Acromegaly. In: Harris GW, Donovan BT, eds. *The pituitary gland.* London: Butterworths, 1966:439–69.

71. Bengtsson BA, Eden S, Ernest I, Oden A, Sjögren B. Epidemiology and long-term survival in acromegaly. *Acta Med Scand* 1988;223:327–35.

72. Etxabe J, Gazambide S, Latorre P, Vazquez JA. Acromegaly: an epidemiological study. *J Endocrinol Invest* 1993;16:181–7.

73. Alexander L, Appleton D, Hall R, Ross WM, Wilkinson R. Epidemiology of acromegaly in the Newcastle region. *Clin Endocrinol* 1980;12:71–9.

74. Barzilay J, Heatley GJ, Cushing GW. Benign and malignant tumors in patients with acromegaly. *Arch Intern Med* 1991;151:1629–32.

75. Ron E, Gridley G, Hrubec Z, Page W, Arona S, Fraumeni JF. Acromegaly and gastrointestinal cancer. *Cancer* 1991;68:1673–7.

76. Ezzat S, Strom C, Melmed S. Colon polyps in acromegaly. *Ann Intern Med* 1991;114:754–5.

77. Terzolo M, Tappero G, Borretta G, et al. High prevalence of colonic polyps in patients with acromegaly. *Arch Intern Med* 1994;154:1272–6.

78. Klein I. Acromegaly and cancer. *Ann Intern Med* 1984;101:706–7.

79. Leavitt J, Klein I, Kendricks F, Galaver J, van Theil DH. Skin tags: a cutaneous marker for colonic polyps. *Ann Intern Med* 1983;98:928–30.

80. Pines A, Rozen P, Ron E, Gilat T. Gastrointestinal tumors in acromegalic patients. *Am J Gastroenterol* 1985;80:266–9.

81. Raymond JM, Lefort G, Sangalli F, et al. Prevalence accrue des polyadenomes recto-colique chez les patients atteints d'acromegalie. Resultats preliminaires chez 15 patients. *Gastroenterol Clin Biol* 1989;13:517.

82. Ituarte EA, Petrini J, Hershman J. Acromegaly and colon cancer. *Ann Intern Med* 1984;101:627–8.
83. Ziel FH, Peters AL. Acromegaly and gastrointestinal adenocarcinomas. *Ann Intern Med* 1989;109:514–5.
84. Brunner JE, Johnson CC, Zafar S, Peterson EL, Brunner JF, Mellinger RC. Colon cancer and polyps in acromegaly: increased risk with family history of colon cancer. *Clin Endocrinol* 1990; 32:65–71.
85. Ezzat S, Melmed S. Are patients with acromegaly at increased risk for neoplasia? *J Clin Endocrinol Metab* 1991;72:245–9.
86. Delhougne B, Deneux C, Abs R, et al. The prevalence of colonic polyps in acromegaly: a colonoscopic and pathological study in 103 patients. *J Clin Endocrinol Metab* 1995;80:3223–6.
87. Moon HD, Simpson ME, Li CH, Evans HM. Neoplasms in rats treated with pituitary growth hormone I. Pulmonary and lymphatic tissues. *Cancer Res* 1950;10:297–308.
88. Halse J, Haugen HN. Calcium and phosphate metabolism in acromegaly. *Acta Endocrinol* 1980;94:459–67.
89. Ieki Y, Miyakoshi H, Nagai Y, et al. The frequency and mechanics of urolithiasis in acromegaly. *Folia Endocrinol Japanica* 1991;67: 755–63.
90. Ho KY, Weissberger AJ. The antinatriuretic action of biosynthetic human growth hormone in man involves activation of the renin-angiotensin system. *Metabolism* 1990;39:133.
91. Lund B, Eskildsen PC, Lund B, Norman AW, Sorensen OH. Calcium and vitamin D metabolism in acromegaly. *Acta Endocrinol* 1981;96:444–50.
92. Caverzasio J, Montessuit C, Bonjour JP. Stimulatory effect of insulin-like growth factor-I on renal Pi transport and plasma 1,25-dihydroxyvitamin D3. *Endocrinol* 1990;127:453–9.
93. Bijlsma JWJ, Nortier JWR, Duursma SA, Croughs RJM, Bosch R, Thijssen JHH. Changes in bone metabolism during treatment of acromegaly. *Acta Endocrinol* 1983;104:153–9.
94. Aloia J, Powell D, Mendizibal E, Roginsky M. Parathyroid function in acromegaly. *Horm Res* 1975;6:145–9.
95. Fredstorp L, Pernow Y, Werner S. The short and long-term effects of octreotide on calcium homeostasis in patients with acromegaly. *Clin Endocrinol* 1993;39:331–6.
96. Takamoto S, Tsuchiya H, Onishi T, et al. Changes in calcium homeostasis in acromegaly treated by pituitary adenomectomy. *J Clin Endocrinol Metab* 1985;61:7–11.
97. Pines A, Olchovsky D. Urolithiasis in acromegaly. *Urology* 1985;26:240–2.
98. Ng LL, Evans DJ. Leucocyte sodium transport in acromegaly. *Clin Endocrinol* 1987;26:471.
99. Ho KY, Kelly JJ. Role of growth hormone in fluid homeostasis. *Horm Res* 1991;36(suppl 1):44–88.
100. Cheek DB, Hill DE. Effect of growth hormone on cell and somatic growth. In: Greep RO, Astwood EB, eds. *Handbook of Physiology.* Vol. 4. Washington, DC: American Physiological Society, 1987: 159–85.
101. McLellan A, Beastall GH, Connell JMC. Body composition and serum growth hormone in treated acromegaly. *J Endocrinol* 1987; 112(suppl):185.
102. Bengtsson BÅ, Brummer RJM, Eden S, Bosaeus I. Body composition in acromegaly. *Clin Endocrinol* 1989;30:121–30.
103. Bengtsson BÅ, Brummer RJ, Eden S, Bosaeus I, Lindstedt G. Body composition in acromegaly: the effect of treatment. *Clin Endocrinol* 1989;31:481–90.
104. McLellan AR, Connell JMC, Beastall GH, Teasdale G, Davies DL. Growth hormone, body composition and somatomedin C after treatment of acromegaly. *Q J Med* 1988;69:997–1008.
105. Hansen TB, Gram J, Bjerre P, Hagen C, Bollerslev J. Body composition in active acromegaly during treatment with octreotide: a double-blind, placebo-controlled cross-over study. *Clin Endocrinol* 1994; 41:323–9.
106. O'Sullivan AJ, Kelly JJ, Hoffman DM, Baxter RC, Ho KKY. Energy metabolism and substrate oxidation in acromegaly. *J Clin Endocrinol Metab* 1995;80:486–91.
107. Grunstein RR, Ho KKY, Sullivan CE. Sleep apnea in acromegaly. *Ann Intern Med* 1991;115:527–32.
108. Grunstein RR, Ho KY, Berthon-Jones M, Stewart D, Sullivan CE. Central sleep apnea is associated with increased ventilatory response to carbon dioxide and hypersecretion of growth hormone in patients with acromegaly. *Am J Resp Crit Care Med* 1994;150:496–502.
109. Grunstein RR, Ho KKY, Sullivan CE. Effect of octreotide, a somatostatin analog, on sleep apnea in patients with acromegaly. *Ann Intern Med* 1994;121:478–83.
110. Issa FG, Sullivan CE. Reversal of central sleep apnea using nasal CPAP. *Chest* 1986;90:165–71.
111. Astrom C, Trojaborg W. Effect of growth hormone on human sleep energy. *Clin Endocrinol* 1992;36:241–5.
112. Astrom C, Christensen L, Gjerris F, Trojaborg W. Sleep in acromegaly before and after treatment with adenomectomy. *Neuroendocrinology* 1991;53:328–31.
113. Pelttari L, Polo O, Rauhala E, et al. Nocturnal breathing abnormalities in acromegaly after adenomectomy. *Clin Endocrinol* 1995;43: 175–82.
114. Cushing H. Psychiatric disturbances associated with ductless glands. *Am J Insanity* 1913;69:965–90.
115. Bleuler M. The psychopathology of acromegaly. *J Nerv Ment Dis* 1951;113:497–511.
116. Abed RT, Clark J, Elbadawy MHF, Cliffe MJ. Psychiatric morbidity in acromegaly. *Acta Psychiatr Scand* 1987;75:635–63.
117. Sablowski N, Pawlik K, Lüdecke DK, Herrmann HD. Aspects of personality change in patients with pituitary adenomas. *Acta Neurochir* 1986;83:8–11.
118. Richert S, Eversmann T, Fahlbusch R, Lierheimer A, Strauss A. Psychopathology, mental functions and personality in patients with acromegaly. *Acta Endocrinol* 1983;253(suppl.):33.
119. Ezzat S. Living with acromegaly. *Endocrinol Metab Clin North Am* 1992;21:753–60.
120. Molitch ME. Clinical manifestations of acromegaly. *Endocrinol Metab Clin North Am* 1992;21:597–614.

CHAPTER 5

Diagnosis of Acromegaly

In many patients, acromegaly is diagnosed on the basis of clinical signs and symptoms (Figs. 36, 37). Confirmation of the diagnosis involves demonstration of biochemical abnormalities of growth hormone (GH) secretion. Pituitary imaging and function tests are also performed to determine the size of the adenoma and to identify possible impairment of hypophyseal function. Because of the anatomic location of the pituitary, ophthalmologic evaluations must also be performed.

CLINICAL DIAGNOSIS

In a certain proportion of patients, the diagnosis can be made at first glance from the characteristic appearance. This subgroup usually has advanced disease, although with increasing awareness of acromegaly, it can be hoped that earlier diagnosis will be achieved. As a consequence of this, a higher index of clinical suspicion will be required, combining classical clinical diagnosis and the

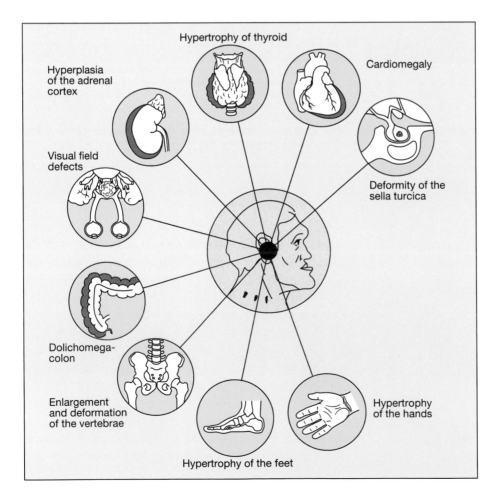

FIG. 36. Clinical features of acromegaly.

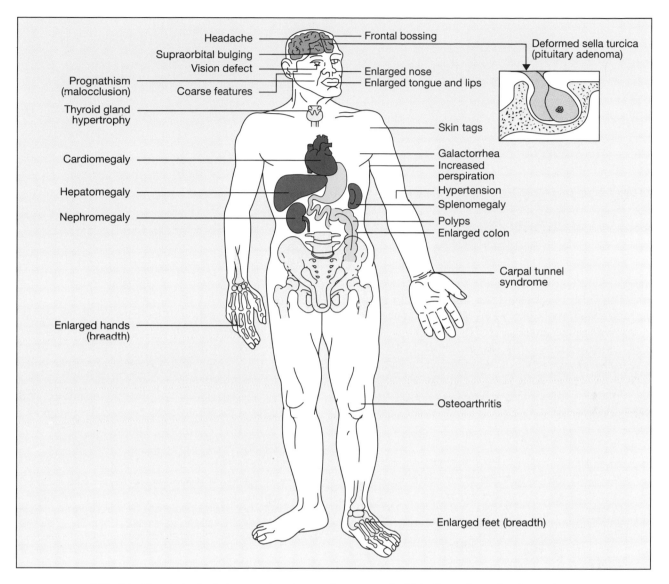

FIG. 37. Morphological changes in advanced acromegaly. Note the enlarged sella turcica.

use of biochemical tests to confirm suspected cases of acromegaly.

The clinical findings include signs of soft-tissue swelling and bone overgrowth, coarsening of facial features, and enlargement of the nose and the supraorbital and nuchal ridges (Figs. 31, 33, 38, 39). Malocclusion is caused by overgrowth of the frontal, nasal, and malar bones and by prognathism (Fig. 32). Dentists need to be aware of acromegaly because it is occasionally diagnosed during dental treatment. Progressively and chronically ill-fitting dentures may be a complaint of acromegalic patients, and is caused by gradual changes in jaw structure. The hands and feet increase in breadth as the skin becomes thickened by soft-tissue swelling (Fig. 40) (acromegalic hands have been described as "spadelike" in appearance). Patients may com-

plain that rings become too tight (Fig. 41) and that their shoe or glove size increases regularly, an abnormal symptom in adults. Ligaments undergo increased collagen synthesis and become destabilized, which becomes clinically apparent as joint hyperlaxity (Fig. 42).

It should be borne in mind that acromegaly is usually insidious in onset and slow to progress. Figure 43 shows the gradual facial changes in an acromegalic patient over a period of 30 years, and examination of earlier photographs of a patient may reveal that the disease has been present for many years before the diagnosis is suspected.

Dorsal kyphosis of the spine not only causes physical deformity but also aggravates cardiovascular and respiratory morbidity (Fig. 44).

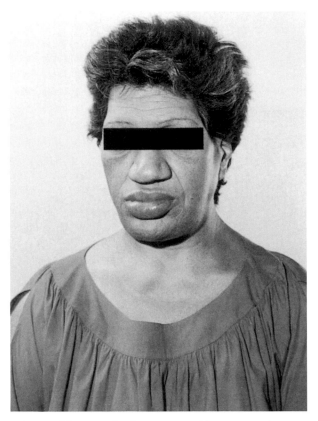

FIG. 38. Photograph of a woman with acromegaly.

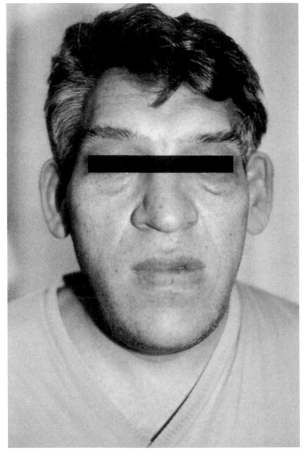

FIG. 39. The acromegalic facies. This is characterized by prognathism, coarse features, and prominent supra- and suborbital ridges. The nasal and the auricular cartilage are thickened and the tongue enlarged. (Courtesy of A. Beckers and A. Stevenaert, University of Liege, Belgium.)

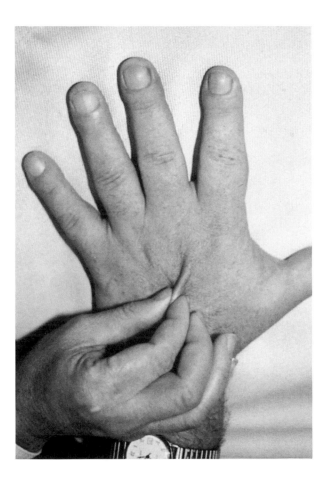

FIG. 40. Assessment of thickness of the skinfold on the dorsum of an acromegalic's hand. (Courtesy of A. Beckers and A. Stevenaert, University of Liege, Belgium.)

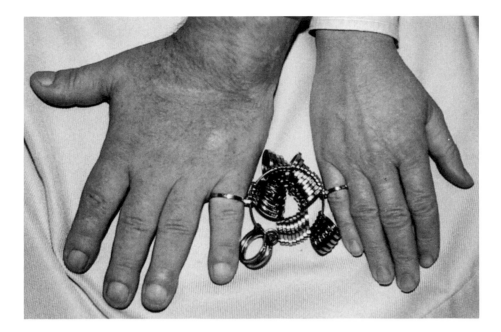

FIG. 41. Changes in finger size can be assessed with jeweller's rings. (Courtesy of A. Beckers and A. Stevenaert, University of Liege, Belgium.)

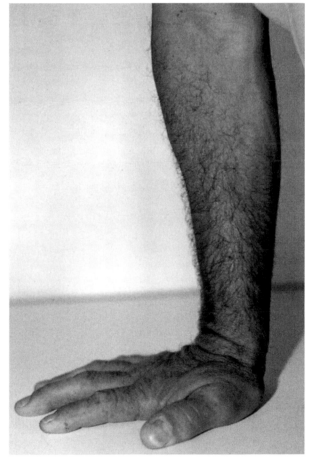

FIG. 42. Ligament hyperlaxity in an acromegalic patient. (Courtesy of A. Beckers and A. Stevenaert, University of Liege, Belgium.)

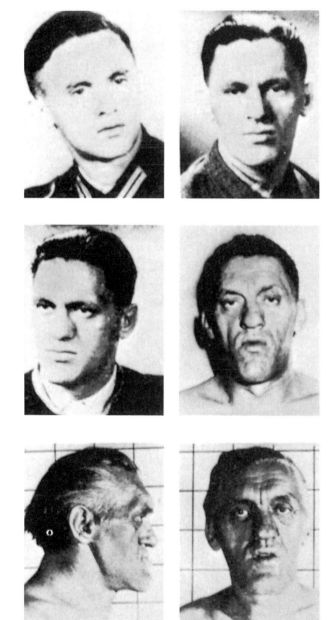

FIG. 43. Morphological changes in the facies of a patient with active acromegaly, over a period of more than 30 years. (From P.H. Althoff with permission.)

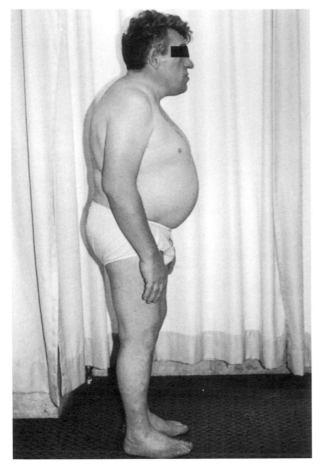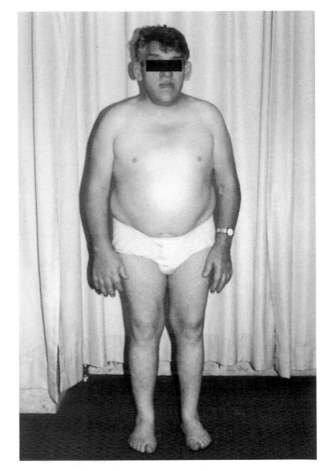

FIG. 44. Long-standing acromegaly results in serious disfigurement. Note the patient's large hands and feet as well as skeletal deformities. (Courtesy of A. Beckers and A. Stevenaert, University of Liege, Belgium.)

BIOCHEMICAL EVALUATION

Basal Tests

Serum Growth Hormone

Random GH measurements have a limited role in the diagnosis of acromegaly (and in follow-up treatment) because of the pulsatility of GH secretion (Fig. 45). However, because GH does not fall to the limit of detectability in acromegaly, the finding of an undetectable GH concentration in a patient suspected of having acromegaly tends to exclude the diagnosis. Indeed, serum GH levels should normally be undetectable in 75% of blood samples obtained through an indwelling venous catheter over a 24-h period. In acromegalics, GH levels are detectable in the majority of blood samples in a 24-h period, usually ranging from 5 μg/L to hundreds of micrograms per liter. Ideally, for GH sampling to be reliable, it should be performed over 24 h. Unfortunately, this is not feasible in many hospitals, so an 8-h sampling time is employed. It should be emphasized that in early acromegaly, clinically relevant disease may occur with GH levels persistently below 2.5 μg/L through-

out the day. Overall, it is best not to rely on GH levels alone, but to employ either plasma IGF-I levels or a dynamic test of GH function, such as an oral glucose tolerance test (OGTT).

Serum Insulin-Like Growth Factor-I

Insulin-like growth factor-I (IGF-I) is a growth hormone-dependent peptide produced by peripheral tissues, which can be measured accurately by a highly specific radioimmunoassay. Because of the fluctuations in GH secretion and the short plasma half-life of GH (c. 20 min), serum IGF-I measurement is more practical for detecting acromegaly. Moreover, various studies have established a very strong correlation between integrated GH secretion over a 24-h period and plasma IGF-I. However, IGF-I concentrations may be elevated in physiologic conditions such as puberty or pregnancy. IGF-I in plasma is largely bound to specific binding proteins, so that conditions causing hypoproteinemia (e.g., advanced hepatic cirrhosis, malnutrition, or nephrotic syndrome) may alter total IGF-I concentrations in a conventional assay. The most widely used assays employ a primary step that removes the binding pro-

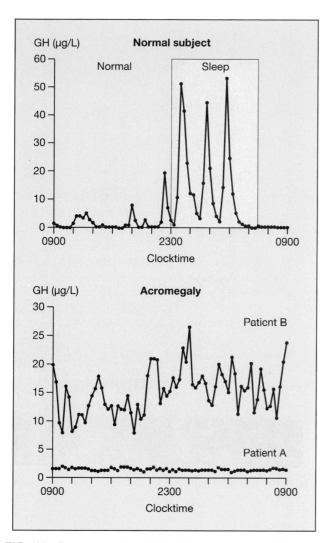

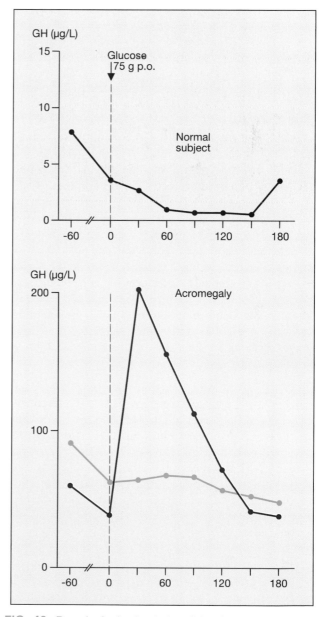

Dynamic Tests

Oral Glucose Tolerance Test

In the normal subject, serum GH levels are suppressed to a nadir of <2 μg/L (or to below the threshold of detectability) after administration of an oral load of glucose (75–100 g). However, in acromegaly GH is not suppressed in this way. Moreover, in some patients GH levels remain unchanged or even rise (Fig. 46). Most physicians are aware of the OGTT from the management of diabetes mellitus, and this test is quite easy to administer in the clinical setting. The OGTT is the most reliable dynamic test now available for confirming the diagnosis of active acromegaly.

FIG. 45. Representative 24 h GH secretory profiles from two patients with acromegaly (lower panel) and from a normal subject (upper panel). Note the blunting of the pulsatile pattern of GH secretion, the failure of GH to fall to an undetectable level and the absence of sleep-entrained GH release in the acromegalic patient whereas patient B shows anarchic bursts of GH. (Courtesy of K.Y. Ho, Garvin Institute of Medical Research, Sydney, Australia.)

teins from the sample, enabling total IGF-I to be assessed. The interpretation of results should be based on a range defined for a particular age group, since IGF-I concentrations show a significant decline with age (1).

Plasma Growth Hormone-Releasing Hormone

Growth hormone-releasing hormone (GHRH) assays are usually of very limited value in the diagnosis of acromegaly, because GH and IGF-I assays are reliable and cost-effective, when used appropriately. Circulating GHRH radioimmunoassays are helpful in identifying those very rare patients in whom acromegaly is caused by ectopic GHRH production or oversecretion of GHRH by the hypothalamus.

FIG. 46. Paradoxical stimulation (black) or non-response (blue) of GH secretion following a 75 g oral glucose load in acromegalic patients.

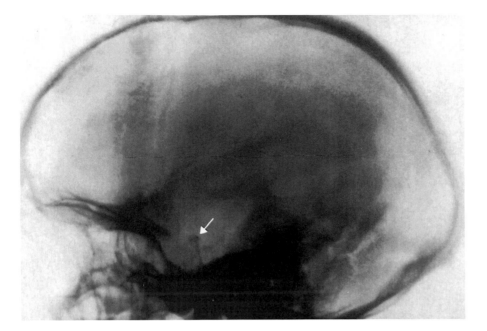

FIG. 47. Lateral skull radiograph shows an enlarged sella turcica.

Thyrotropin-Releasing Hormone and Gonadotropin-Releasing Hormone Tests

Neither administration of thyrotropin-releasing hormone (TRH) nor of gonadotropin-releasing hormone (GnRH) alters GH secretion in normal individuals. Patients with active acromegaly exhibit a paradoxical rise in serum GH levels in 25% of cases, although a lack of response (i.e., a normal response) is seen in 50% of patients. The use of paradoxical GH responses to these TRH/GnRH dynamic tests are not recommended as diagnostic end points because they lack specificity. GH responses are not seen in all patients with acromegaly and may occur in generalized conditions other than acromegaly, such as growth phase puberty, diabetes mellitus anorexia nervosa starvation, and chronic renal failure.

Radiologic Evaluation

X-Ray

Lateral plain skull radiography (Figs. 47–49) has been used for many years to assess the state of the sella turcica and other typical bony changes (prognathism, enlargement of sinuses) in patients with suspected acromegaly. Although this method is very inexpensive, it provides no information regarding soft-tissue changes or the size of the pituitary adenoma. In addition, interpretation of these films is quite prone to error and is associated with very high false-positive rates, especially in the hands of an inexperienced radiologist. Therefore, x-ray has been supplanted by computed tomography (CT scan) and magnetic resonance imaging (MRI).

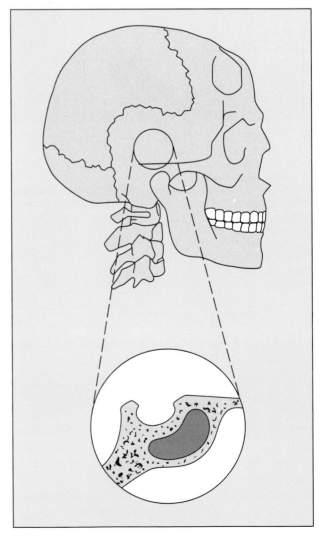

FIG. 48. Plain skull radiography of a normal subject.

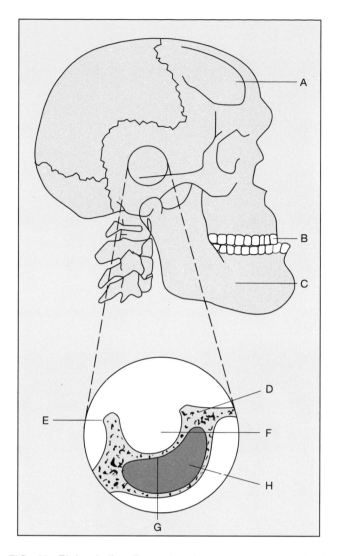

FIG. 49. Plain skull radiography of an acromegalic patient. A, Hypertrophy of the frontal sinuses; B, malocclusion; C, prognathism; D/E, tendency towards vertical alignment of the anterior and posterior walls of the sella turcica (erosion of the clinoid process; F, enlargement of the sella turcica; G, depression of the floor of the sella turcica; H, sphenoidal sinus.

Computed Tomography

High-resolution CT imaging of the pituitary and suprasellar region, particularly with the use of i.v. contrast media, have made it possible to demonstrate the pituitary tumor and the extent of any suprasellar extension (Fig. 50). The usual axial view is supplemented by coronal high-resolution CT scans, which can demonstrate tumors as small as 3–4 mm in diameter. Dynamic angioscan to demonstrate lateral extensions is an auxiliary method. Pituitary gland height provides a good single measure for the evaluation of pituitary size.

Magnetic Resonance Imaging

MRI has added a new dimension to the delineation of tumor and its surrounding soft-tissue structures. It provides better definition than CT of the suprasellar cisterns, cavernous sinuses, carotid arteries, pituitary stalk, and optic tracts (Figs. 51–53). This information is of particular interest to the surgeon because a planned approach may need to be modified to clear all tumor tissue that has extended into the cavernous sinuses and other structures. Intraoperative MRI may become standard in the future which will enable the surgeon to evaluate rapidly the extent of tumor removal while the operative field is still accessible. The contrast agent, gadolinium-DTPA achieves improved contrast between the adenoma and surrounding normal tissues. In a chronic condition such as acromegaly, which requires regular evaluation before and after treatment, MRI is the safest and most effective radiologic procedure, as patients are not repeatedly exposed to ionizing radiation.

Positron Emission Tomography

Positron emission tomography (PET) is an imaging technique that allows in vivo visualization and quantitative determination of functional and biochemical parameters of pituitary tumor activity. With this technique, dopamine D_2-receptor binding and increased amino acid metabolism can be measured using C-L methionine, which reflects tumor activity of pituitary adenomas. However, PET is not widely used at present, being limited to specialist and academic centers, and therefore its value in the clinical setting remains to be determined.

Single Photon Emission Computed Tomography

Single photon emission computed tomography (SPECT), in contrast to conventional nuclear medicine imaging methods, provides three-dimensional images of the concentration of a radiopharmaceutical agent within an organ. Major advances have been made in this field, many of which have occurred as an offshoot of the development of the somatostatin analogue octreotide. By conjugating octreotide with DTPA, radiolabeled indium [^{111}In] can be attached, to form a compound known as [^{111}In]DTPA-octreotide or [^{111}In] pentetreotide (available commercially as OctreoScan, Mallinkrodt, St. Louis, MO, U.S.A.).

This complex retains the binding capability of octreotide to somatostatin receptors and allows scintigraphic visualization of sites with high receptor densities. Krenning and colleagues (2) at the University of Rotterdam, Holland, have pioneered this technique. GH-producing pituitary adenomas have been shown to contain specific binding sites for somatostatin, mainly subtypes 2 and 5 (3), although subtype 1 has also been reported (4). With this in mind, it is

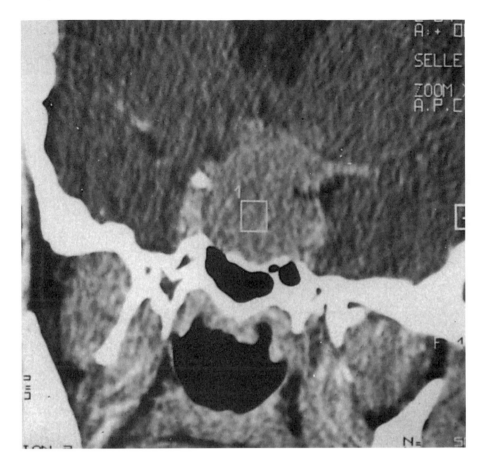

FIG. 50. CT scan of an acromegalic patient demonstrating a large pituitary tumor with suprasellar extension. (Courtesy of J.P. Tauber, University of Toulouse, France.)

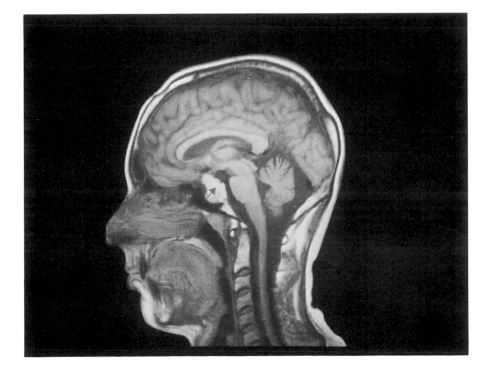

FIG. 51. Sagittal magnetic resonance imaging (MRI) showing a pituitary tumor in a 28-year-old male acromegalic. (Courtesy of P.O. Lundberg, C. Muhr and M. Bergstrom, University of Uppsala, Sweden.)

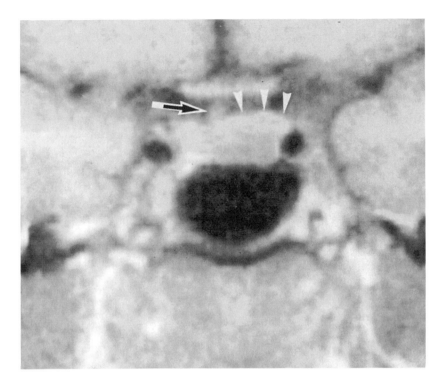

FIG. 52. Magnetic resonance imaging (MRI) of the sella turcica in an acromegalic patient. Non-enhanced frontal T1-weighted image (TR = 520 ms; TE = 15 ms). Bulging of the sellar diaphragm with displacement of the pituitary stalk to the right.

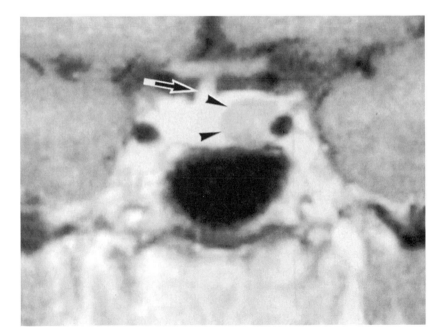

FIG. 53. Frontal T1-weighted image (TR = 520 ms; TE = 15 ms) after i.v. injection of Gadolinium-Dota at a dosage of 0.1 mmol per kg. Clearly delineated adenoma. Note displacement of the contrast-enhanced pituitary stalk. (Courtesy of G. Wilms, G. Marchal, A. Baert and R. Bouillon, Catholic University of Louvain, Belgium.)

possible to locate accurately pituitary adenomas that express somatostatin receptors (Fig. 54). This enables precise identification of the size of the pituitary adenoma and any degree of local extension, which may be extremely helpful in future planning of surgical adenoma resection. In addition, ectopic lesions that secrete GHRH (e.g., bronchial carcinoids) can be localized if they express somatostatin receptors for which octreotide has high affinity (subtypes 2, 3, and 5). Although it is believed that this technique holds out promise as a possible method of selecting patients for successful treatment with long-acting somatostatin analogues (5), normal pituitary cells express somatostatin receptors, thereby making the specificity of such a test uncertain.

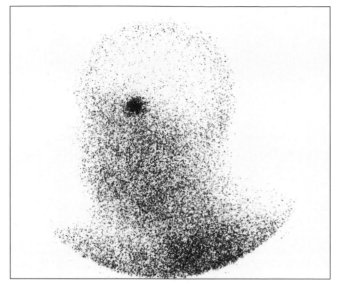

FIG. 54. [¹¹¹In]DTPA octreotide scintigraphy (OctreoScan) (24 h after injection of 200 MBq) of an acromegalic patient showing on a left lateral view the accumulation of radiolabeled octreotide in a GH-secreting pituitary adenoma. (Courtesy of E.P. Krenning, University of Rotterdam, The Netherlands.)

DIFFERENTIAL DIAGNOSIS

As befits a rare condition like acromegaly, few conditions mimic the disease. However, five conditions do exist that may present in a manner similar to acromegaly:

1. Multiple endocrine neoplasia type I (MEN-I). This is a syndrome characterized by a pattern of endocrine-active tumors, including pituitary adenomas. In patients who have close relatives with acromegaly (familial acromegaly), MEN-I must be ruled out. The coexistence of parathyroid or islet-cell neoplasms points strongly to the presence of MEN-I.

2. Hypothyroidism induces changes in features, skin and voice which may be suggestive of acromegaly in some cases, although this can be easily ruled out with thyroid function tests.

3. A rare familial condition known as pachydermoperiostosis, can be mistaken for acromegaly, as it is characterized by coarsening of facial features, thickened skin and hypertrophic osteoarthropathy. The clinical resemblance to acromegaly is not reflected by abnormal GH levels, dynamic function tests and radiological evidence.

4. A small number of patients have been reported to have acromegalic features in the absence of overt GH and IGF-I abnormalities, a condition known as acromegaloidism. These patients may have a defect in ligand-receptor binding or signaling.

5. A rare condition known as McCune-Albright syndrome can confuse the diagnosis of acromegaly. This disease is characterized by a triad of clinical findings: polyostotic fibrous dysplasia, café-au-lait spots and sexual precocity. These patients may also suffer from other endocrine diseases, including acromegaly. In McCune-Albright syndrome, the radiologic bony changes are not what would be expected in classical acromegaly, and pituitary abnormalities may not be noticeable. Prolactin hypersecretion is commonly found in this syndrome (80%), compared with 30% in acromegaly. Differentiation between these two conditions should be made on history and physical examination (looking for the classic triad above). This can be confirmed by thorough radiological surveys and analysis of biopsied bony lesions.

REFERENCES

1. Daughaday WH. A personal history of the origin of the somatomedin hypothesis and recent challenges to its validity. *Perspect Biol Med* 1994;32:194–211.
2. Krenning EP, Kwekkeboom DJ, Bakker WH, et al. Somatostatin receptor scintigraphy with [¹¹¹In-DTPA-D-Phe¹]- and [¹²³I-Tyr³]-octreotide: the Rotterdam experience with more than 1000 patients. *Eur J Nucl Med* 1993;20:716–31.
3. Greenman Y, Melmed S. Heterogenous expression of two somatostatin receptor subtypes in pituitary tumors. *J Clin Endocrinol Metab* 1994;78:398.
4. Miller GM, Alexander JM, Bikkal HA, Katznelson L, Zervas NT, Klibanski A. Somatostatin receptor subtype gene expression in pituitary adenomas. *J Clin Endocrinol Metab* 1995;80:1386–92.
5. Reubi JC, Landolt AM. The growth hormone responses to octreotide in acromegaly correlate with adenoma somatostatin receptor status. *J Clin Endocrinol Metab* 1989;68:844–50.

CHAPTER 6

Treatment of Acromegaly

The main aims of therapy are to improve clinical symptoms, normalize GH/IGF-I secretion, and reduce tumor mass, without compromising anterior pituitary function (Fig. 55). Although effective management may reverse clinical abnormalities and restore normal endocrine function, a "cure" for acromegaly is often difficult to achieve, because active disease has been reported in patients with well-suppressed GH/IGF-I. Moreover, with stricter criteria for biochemical normalization being set, it will probably become less common in the future for effective disease control to be brought about using only a single therapeutic option.

BIOCHEMICAL NORMALIZATION CRITERIA

The question of what constitutes normal growth hormone secretion is of paramount importance when the success of therapy is evaluated (Fig. 56). Unfortunately, a simple definition is not possible in view of the pulsatile nature of GH secretion and the wide variations in individual secretory patterns. Many series have arbitrarily defined normalization as a random GH concentration of <5 μg/L but do not present 24-h integrated GH levels. Other studies provide only mean percentage falls in GH levels. This is understandable, given the difficulty of performing 24-h serum collections in the busy clinical setting. Random GH levels are not reliable because of the inherent pulsatility and rhythmicity of GH secretion. If a 24-h GH collection is not practical, an 8-h collection may provide a reasonable alternative. Serum IGF-I levels do not vary greatly on a day-to-day basis and therefore provide an accurate reflection of the patient's true biochemical status. IGF-I levels should be corrected for age- and sex-related variations.

One possible approach is to define normalization in quantitative or qualitative terms, or to use circulating IGF-I concentrations as an index of the biologic activity of GH. Therefore, a quantitative assessment of normal GH secretion is obtained by defining normal output in terms of mean 24-h (or 8-h) GH concentrations. This requires detailed 24-h GH measurements in normal subjects to establish the normal range. Ho et al. (1) reported that the normal range for mean 24-h GH secretion was 2.2 μg/L and for IGF-I 0.4–1.6 U/ml in adults. Newer chemiluminescence assays are expected to lower the criteria for normalization even further, as Chapman et al. (2) have shown normal men and women to have nadir GH concentrations after a glucose load of 0.057 μg/L and 0.71 μg/L, respectively. This indicates that the strictest criteria for GH normalization are warranted.

A qualitative approach is to define normality as the complete restoration of the normal circadian properties of GH secretion, such as the attainment of undetectable nadir, sleep-triggered release of GH, and a pattern in which nocturnal output exceeds daytime output (absence of the paradoxical GH responses to provocative stimuli) (Fig. 57).

Clearly, the ideal treatment should suppress GH to undetectable levels for 75% of the 24-h period, with concomitant normalization of IGF-I levels. Failure to achieve these criteria implies "control" or "remission" rather than "cure" of acromegaly. Clinical judgment is required in marginal cases where GH is normal and IGF-I is slightly or moderately elevated. The burden of additional treatment (e.g., three daily injections of octreotide) must be balanced against the possible reduction in morbidity and mortality afforded by the strictest biochemical control.

Normalization of GH

Reduction of pituitary tumour mass

Correction of visual and neurological complications

Preservation of pituitary function

Prevention of biochemical or local recurrence

FIG. 55. Therapeutic aims of treating acromegaly.

Criteria	Definition of normal
Quantitative GH IGF₁	mean 24h GH in range of age-matched normal subjects IGF₁ in range of age-matched normal subjects
Qualitative 24h secretory pattern	undetectable nadir sleep entrained release, greater nocturnal release
Dynamic testing Oral glucose tolerance test	resolution of paradoxical responses

FIG. 56. Criteria of normalization of GH secretion in assessing the outcome of therapy in acromegaly.

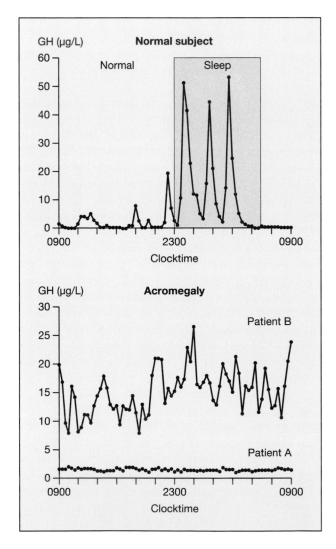

FIG. 57. Representative 24-h GH secretory profiles from two patients with acromegaly (lower panel) and from a normal subject (upper panel). Note the blunting of the pulsatile pattern of GH secretion, the failure of GH to fall to an undetectable level and the absence of sleep-entrained GH release in acromegalic patient A whereas patient B shows anarchic bursts of GH. (Courtesy of K.Y. Ho.)

TREATMENT MODALITIES

Surgery

Surgery, developed by Cushing (3) in the early decades of the 20th century, was the first effective treatment for acromegaly. The transsphenoidal approach to removing the pituitary adenoma is the method of choice in the majority of patients (Figs. 58–60). Tumors that have invaded the cavernous sinus and are not amenable to either transsphenoidal resection or radiotherapy have been removed successfully via a transcranial or transcavernous approach (4,5). Surgery is successful in about 75% of patients with microadenomas (<10 mm) that show no evidence of local invasion (6), and is successful (GH <5 μg/L) in approximately 60–65% of cases overall [Fig. 61 (7–15) and Fig. 62 (11, 12, 16–18)]. Normal pituitary function may be maintained in these cases, especially if the tumor is well encapsulated. The initial drop in GH secretion may be quite dramatic but actual cure is rarely achieved and, despite the excellence of modern neurosurgical techniques, the long-term outcome is somewhat disappointing. Ross and Wilson (12) reviewed results of transsphenoidal surgery in 214 of their own patients and 1,360 patients from 30 surgical series worldwide. Plasma GH dipped below 5 μg/L in 56% of their own patients and in 60% of patients in the other series. Success rates vary considerably (between 44 and 92%) and appear to depend on the skill of the surgeon, the size and invasiveness of the tumor (microadenomas respond better than macroadenomas), and the biochemical criteria of cure (usually a GH level <5 μg/L). More recent surgical studies have applied a stricter definition of cure, such as GH <2 μg/L alone or 5 μg/L with normalization of IGF-1 levels (2.2 U/ml). Remission rates in these series vary between 51.7 and 76.2% (14,15).

Acromegaly may recur several years after surgery despite "normal" postoperative GH levels (<5 μg/L or <10 μg/L) and normal dynamic responses (e.g., after oral glucose tolerance testing). Postsurgical relapse may indi-

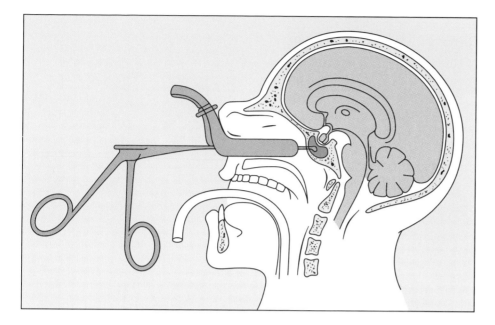

FIG. 58. The transsphenoidal approach in surgery for removal of a pituitary microadenoma. The sphenoid sinus is reached by the transnasal route, and the floor of the sella and dura are opened, thereby exposing the pituitary.

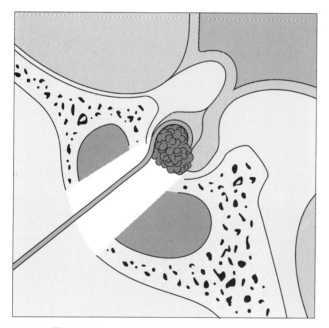

FIG. 59. This approach permits the selective excision of the adenoma (adenomectomy).

cate a recurrent adenoma, incomplete resection of the original adenoma, or invasion of the dura by functioning GH-secreting tumor cell nests that are difficult to visualize and to resect. As an illustration of this last point, Fahlbusch and colleagues (19) reported microinfiltration of the basal dura by tumor cells in 44 of 102 (43%) cases, thereby underscoring the importance of basal dural resection. Second surgery may be necessary but only in patients for whom there is a realistic chance of adequate tumor removal. The success rate for reoperation is no higher than for the initial surgery, and Laws et al. (20) reported that the complication rate was higher in patients undergoing reoperation. Complications of surgery include cerebrospinal fluid leaks, sinusitis, visual damage, hypopituitarism, transient or permanent diabetes insipidus, and meningitis. Ross and Wilson (12) reported a complication rate of approximately 6.7% in their review of over 1,000 transsphenoidal adenomectomies for acromegaly. However, most of these complications are temporary and must be weighed against the immense value of tumor removal and halting active acromegaly.

Radiation Therapy

Radiation was first used as a therapy for acromegaly at approximately the same time as Cushing began surgical treatment of pituitary adenomas (21). Modern radiotherapy relies on linear accelerators or ^{60}Co to produce photons with energies in the million electron volt (MeV) range. The aim of this therapy is to deliver a dose of radiation directly to the tumor that is sufficient to halt division of the adenomatous tissue, thus retarding the hypersecretion of GH. Focusing of the beam must be precise so as to prevent irradiation of vital structures such as healthy pituitary tissue, the hypothalamus, optic nerves, and cerebral cortex. Radiotherapy is suitable for patients who have failed previous surgery or who cannot or are unwilling to undergo tumor resection. A review of the literature shows that approximately 50% of patients are controlled (GH <5 μg/L) 10 years after initiating radiotherapy (Fig. 63) (22–26). It has been noted that patients with lower pretreatment GH levels reached an "acceptable" GH level (<10 μg/L or <20 μg/L) after radiotherapy more rapidly than patients with a high pretreatment GH concentration (27). Although, in a very

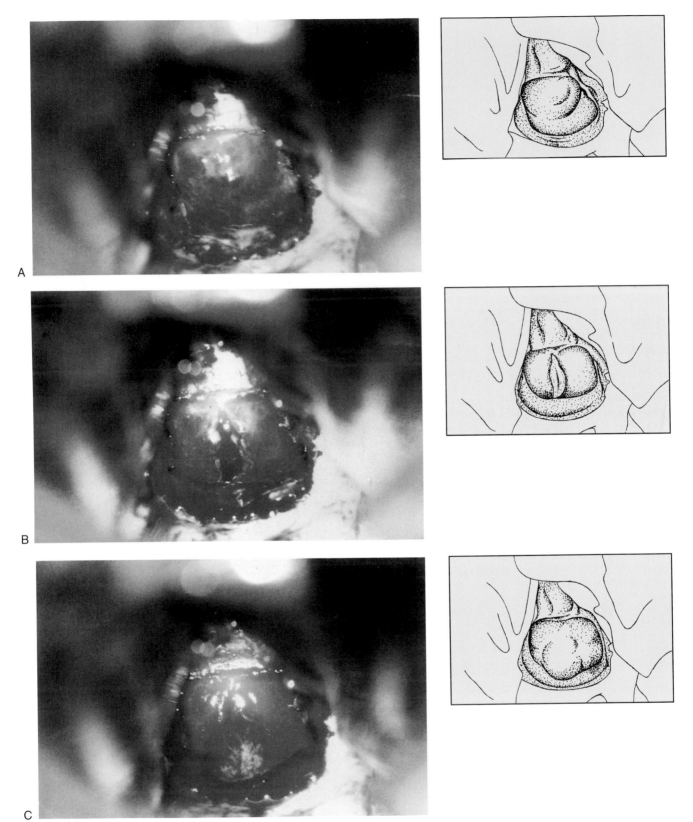

FIG. 60. Stages in transsphenoidal surgery. **(A)** Intact pituitary; **(B)** vertical incision in the anterior hypophysis; **(C)** excision of the adenoma; **(D)** final extraction; **(E)** inspection of the tumor cavity. (Courtesy of A. Stevenaert, University of Liege, Belgium.)

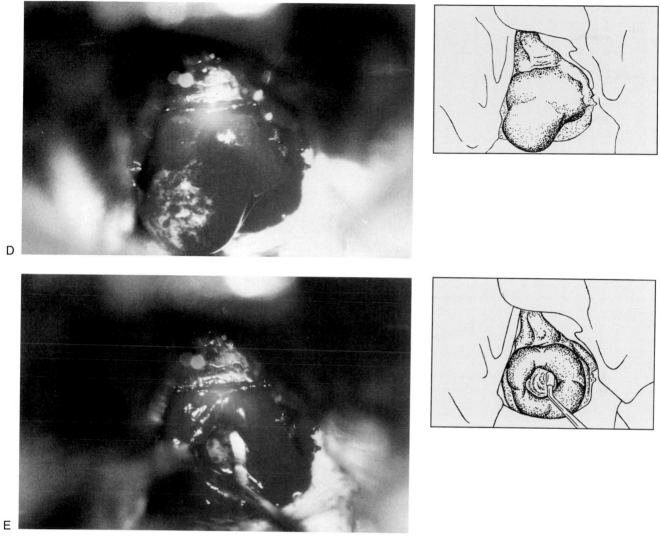

D

E

FIG. 60 *Continued*

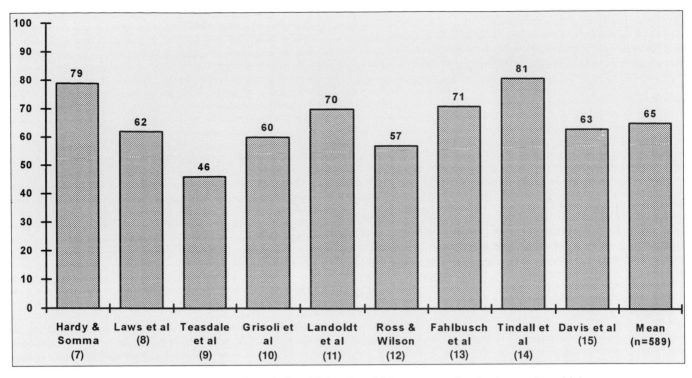

FIG. 61. The percentage rate of remission (GH ≤ 5 μg/L) in acromegaly after transsphenoidal adenomectomy. (Adapted from ref. 19.)

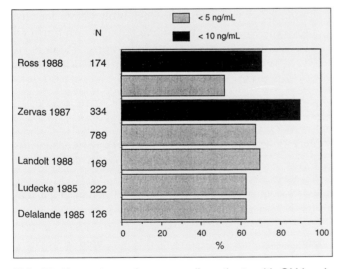

FIG. 62. Percentage of acromegalic patients with GH levels below 5 or 10 ng/ml after transsphenoidal surgery. (From Melmed S, et al. Clinical review 75. Recent advances in pathogenesis, diagnosis, and management of acromegaly. *J Clin Endocrinol Metab* 1995;80:3395–402.)

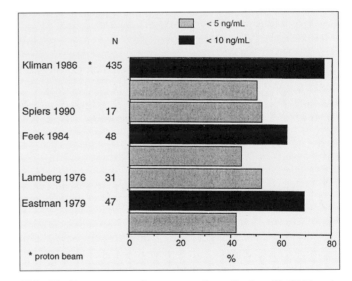

FIG. 63. Percentage of acromegalic patients with GH levels below 5 or 10 ng/ml 10 years after initiating radiotherapy. (From Melmed S, et al. Clinical review 75. Recent advances in pathogenesis, diagnosis, and management of acromegaly. *J Clin Endocrinol Metab* 1995;80:3395–402.)

comprehensive review, Eastman et al. (28) concluded that pretreatment GH had no influence on postradiation biochemical outcome. According to present criteria for biochemical control (GH <2 μg/L or even <1 μg/L), these results do not represent an acceptable level of control. Because the primary goal of treatment is the lowering of

GH and IGF-I levels to the normal range, medical therapy with the somatostatin analogue octreotide or the dopamine agonist bromocriptine should be also be considered for these patients. In the interim between radiotherapy and biochemical improvement, medical therapy with a somatostatin analogue (e.g., octreotide) or a dopamine agonist (see below) should be instituted to avoid the deleterious effects of high GH/IGF-I on life expectancy and morbidity.

The three principal forms of radiotherapy are external x-ray radiation, proton-beam irradiation, and interstitial irradiation. A fourth alternative, stereotactic radiosurgery, has also been developed.

X-Ray Irradiation

Conventional x-ray therapy delivers a total of 4,000–5,000 rads over multiple sessions in period of 4–6 weeks. It is slow to take effect and requires 10 years for 81% of patients to achieve serum GH concentrations below 10 μg/L. Radiotherapy arrests tumor growth immediately in the vast majority of cases, and most adenomas shrink in size. The slow rate of response is the major disadvantage of this treatment, as patients will continue to have unacceptably high levels of GH and IGF-I for several years after treatment.

Proton-Beam Irradiation

The second method, heavy-particle proton-beam therapy, has the advantage of delivering high doses (10,000–15,000 rads) to the pituitary during a single session.

Implantation of a Radiation Source

The third method, intrasellar implantation of yttrium-90 seeds, has a success rate of about 50%. This technique is almost obsolete because, although it is effective, it combines the drawbacks of surgery and radiation.

Stereotactic Radiosurgery

Stereotactic radiosurgery (e.g., γ-knife) involves the delivery of extremely high doses of radiation to a small target area of tumor. This method can achieve complete destruction of the target area in one session, or can allow more gradual treatment if applied in a fractionated manner. Radiosurgery is still limited to a small number of centers worldwide, and it has been suggested that side effects are increased compared to conventional radiotherapy. Further research is obviously required before a final determination can be made regarding the value of γ-knife and other radiosurgical techniques for treatment of acromegaly.

The side effects of irradiation are significant (Table 6). The most common complication is hypopituitarism, which usually becomes manifest years after irradiation has taken place, and many patients require lifelong hormone supplementation. The rank order of sensitivity to radiation-induced hormonal insufficiency is GH > FSH/LH > ACTH > TSH. Another important side effect is visual loss, which has become less common with refinements in tech-

TABLE 6. *Side effects of radiotherapy in acromegaly*
Pituitary hormonal deficits
Hypothyroidism (TSH)
Hypogonadism (FSH/LH)
Hypoadrenalism (ACTH)
Panhypopituitarism
Visual impairment
Chiasmal damage
Optic nerve/tract damage
Necrosis of brain tissue/functional deficits
Brain stem necrosis
Temporal lobe necrosis
Increased risk of brain malignancy
Glioma
Fibrosarcoma
Meningioma (?)

nique and dose reductions. It has been suggested that patients with acromegaly are at greater risk for radiation-induced optic tract damage because of associated vascular disease, although this remains theoretical. Complications such as parasellar radionecrosis with cranial nerve palsy, tumor necrosis with hemorrhage, and apoplexy are thought to occur in 5% of patients. The frequency of these local complications may be higher when proton-beam therapy is employed. Suprasellar tumor extension is therefore a contraindication for heavy-particle therapy. Patients also describe a feeling of lethargy and impaired memory, which may be caused by damage to brain structures such as the temporal lobes. Future MRI studies should help to define the prevalence of this damage.

Finally, concerns have been raised regarding the incidence of second (nonpituitary) malignancy in patients who receive radiotherapy for pituitary adenomas (29). Data from the Royal Marsden Hospital in England have shown that the relative risk for development of a second brain tumor was 9.4 compared with the general population (30,31). Jones (32) has reported a much lower incidence of second tumors, and further studies will be required to define the actual risk posed by radiotherapy in this area.

Medical Therapy

Two classes of drugs are available for treatment of acromegaly, dopamine agonists (e.g., bromocriptine) and somatostatin analogues, such as octreotide. These agents can be very useful in patients who have failed or are unsuitable for surgery and/or radiotherapy (or who are waiting for the effects of radiotherapy to become evident). The development of octreotide has had a great impact on the treatment of acromegaly, and data have now been collected in patients who have been experiencing the beneficial effects of the drug for 14 years.

Somatostatin Analogues

As described in previous chapters, somatostatin and GHRH act together to determine hypothalamic regulation of GH release from the anterior pituitary. Dense concentrations of somatostatin receptors are found on normal pituitary tissue on many GH-secreting pituitary adenomas (33). Somatostatin has a very short plasma half-life (c. 2.5 min) and is associated with rebound hypersecretion of hormones such as GH and glucagon when treatment is halted (34). Therefore, somatostatin is unsuitable as a treatment for reducing GH secretion over the long term. For this reason, a number of long-acting somatostatin analogues have been developed, octreotide (SMS 201-995, Sandostatin®), lanreotide (BIM-23104), and vapreotide (RC-160) (35–37). Of these, only octreotide is registered worldwide for the treatment of acromegaly, and it has been shown to reduce GH/IGF-I levels effectively and to control disease symptoms during long-term treatment.

Octreotide is a cyclic octapeptide that retains the specific amino acid sequence required to bind with high affinity to somatostatin receptors, while its remaining structure is designed to resist enzymatic attack (Fig. 64). Together, these features give octreotide a plasma half-life of almost 2 h, and it suppresses GH with approximately 40-fold greater potency than native somatostatin. It is noteworthy that suppression of GH persists after plasma levels of octreotide have begun to decrease, indicating prolonged receptor occupancy by octreotide (38). In addition, octreotide inhibits insulin secretion significantly less than does

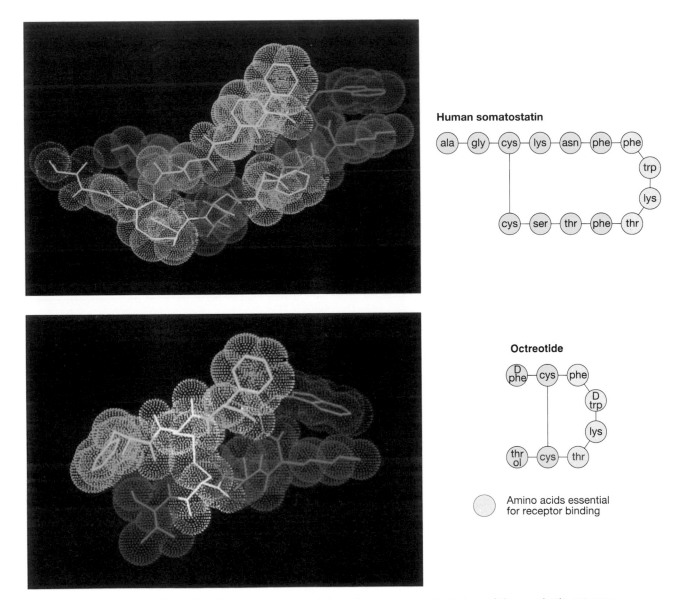

FIG. 64. Three-dimensional surface representation of human somatostatin and the synthetic octapeptide analogue octreotide. (Courtesy of R. Breckenridge.)

glucagon, thereby largely avoiding potential problems with hypoglycemia. Rebound hypersecretion after cessation of octreotide therapy does not occur (39).

Biochemical Effects of Octreotide

Early work demonstrated the efficacy of octreotide in the suppression of GH/IGF-I in acromegalic patients (40). Doses of 50–100 μg of octreotide decreased GH levels by up to 86% over a period of 2–6 h after subcutaneous administration. It was also shown that 100 μg of octreotide provided a significantly longer period of GH suppression than a 50-μg dose. The 50-μg dose of octreotide suppressed GH levels to 62% of pretreatment levels, and the 100-μg dose suppressed GH by 81% 2–10 h after administration. Short-term studies were followed by favorable data on the chronic administration of octreotide in acromegalic patients, in whom the beneficial acute effects were maintained (41,42). Long-term octreotide therapy was found to further decrease GH levels over time. Furthermore, circulating IGF-I concentrations gradually decreased in many patients and were normalized in approximately 50% of patients.

Since the mid-1980s, several large studies have been published regarding the long-term effects of octreotide treatment in acromegaly (43–46) (Fig. 65). Harris et al. (45) reported results of a retrospective case collection of 178 patients at 22 centers worldwide who were treated with 50–1,500 μg s.c. octreotide per day (mean 253 μg/day). In their study, 46% of patients had a GH level <5 μg/L and 20.8% had GH levels ≤2 μg/L. IGF-I concentrations were normalized in 36% of cases. These data were confirmed by a prospective North American placebo-controlled, multicenter trial of octreotide (100 or 250 μg s.c. every 8 h) in 115 acromegalic patients (44). Integrated mean GH levels were reduced to <5 μg/L in 49–53% of patients, and IGF-I levels were normal in 55–68% of patients (Fig. 66). They also found that the higher dose of octreotide (250 μg s.c. every 8 h) did not significantly improve biochemical control. In summary, octreotide (100 μg every 8 h) decreases GH levels to <5 μg/L in approximately 50% of patients, and 85–90% of patients experience a significant decrease in GH secretion. IGF-I levels are also well controlled by octreotide, with normal levels noted in 40–70% of patients treated.

Newman et al. (46) recently reported safety and efficacy data from 103 acromegalic patients treated with octreotide (300–1,500 μg s.c.) for a mean duration of 24 months, most of whom took part in the study reported by Ezzat et al. (44). GH levels fell from 30.9 μg/L to 5.7 μg/L after 3 months and remained suppressed throughout the trial. Plasma IGF-I concentrations were normal at <50% of the assessment periods in 64% of patients treated for 12–30 months. Newman and colleagues (46) noted no evidence of patients developing gradual resistance to octreotide, and tachyphy-

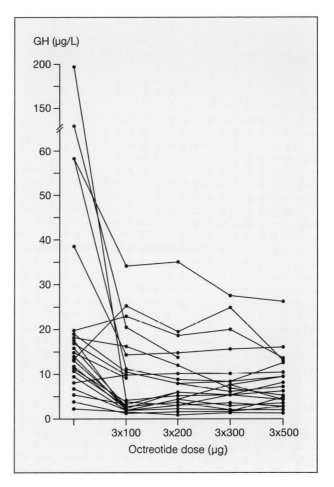

FIG. 65. Effects of incremental doses of octreotide on GH secretion in 29 of the 58 acromegalic patients who received 500 μg t.i.d. [From G. Sassolas et al., 1990 (43) with permission.]

laxis has yet to be reported in patients receiving long-term octreotide.

Consistent GH suppression has also been obtained with a continuous subcutaneous pump infusion of octreotide (47–51). This mode of administration provides consistent GH/IGF-I suppression throughout the day and avoids elevations in GH as octreotide levels fall 6–8 h after injection. Although intermittent s.c. injections of octreotide are the predominant method of administering octreotide, some patients have found the implantable pump useful and highly effective. Concerns were raised that continuously administered octreotide may increase the risk for side effects such as gallstones, compared with the risk for patients receiving intermittent octreotide injections. However, Tauber et al. (52) reported recently that no such risk exists.

Because peptides such as octreotide are rapidly degraded in the gut, an orally administered form does not appear to be feasible. A nasal powder formulation of octreotide has been developed, which has approximately 25% bioavailability via the nasal mucosa (53). A 500-μg dose of nasally administered octreotide has the bioavailability of

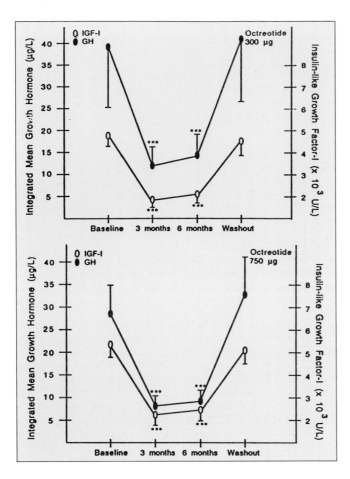

FIG. 66. Effect of low- and high-dose octreotide on integrated growth hormone and insulin-like growth factor-I levels. Integrated mean growth hormone and insulin-like growth factor-I concentrations sampled during 8 h in acromegalic patients treated with subcutaneous octreotide 100 μg every 8 h (n = 50) (top) or 250 μg every 8 h (n = 54) (bottom) for up to 6 months followed by 1 month of washout. ***p <0.001 compared with baseline. (From Ezzat S, et al. Octreotide treatment of acromegaly. A randomized multicenter study. *Ann Intern Med* 1992;117:711–18.)

100 μg of s.c.-injected octreotide, but is not as potent as the injectable form. Octreotide nasal powder is not commercially available.

Because of the lack of a feasible oral formulation and in an effort to improve the convenience of administration, a long-acting repeatable (LAR) depot form of octreotide has been produced. In LAR octreotide, the drug is incorporated into biodegradable DL-lactide-co-glycolide polymer microspheres, which are injected intramuscularly. This reduces GH/IGF-I secretion effectively when it is administered once every 28 days at a dose of 3–30 mg (54–56). Lancranjan and co-workers (55) studied the pharmacology and clinical efficacy of LAR octreotide in 100 acromegalic patients (Figs. 67 and 68). Peak octreotide levels were noted 1 h after intramuscular injection at all doses from 3– 30 mg/day

and serum levels declined to low levels over the following 12 h. At 7 days after injection, serum octreotide levels began to increase and a dose-dependent plateau was reached from day 14 to day 42, which was steady over 12-h observation periods. After day 42 the plateau octreotide concentration decreased gradually, a pattern which the authors believed to favor a once-monthly dosage regimen. The peak–trough octreotide level fluctuations during the plateau phase were on the order of 25%, compared with a variation of up to 200% during standard intermittent s.c. injections. Steady-state concentrations of octreotide were reached after three injections at 28-day intervals and were 1.6 times greater than the initial peak levels seen 1 h after administration of the first dose. Accumulation of octreotide after repeated doses was not noted to any significant degree. GH was persistently suppressed during the plateau phase on days 14–42, and consistent stable inhibition of GH secretion was seen beginning with the third monthly dose of octreotide. In patients who had only a good response to intermittently injected octreotide, 79.5% experienced a drop in GH levels to <2 μg/L, with 67.9%

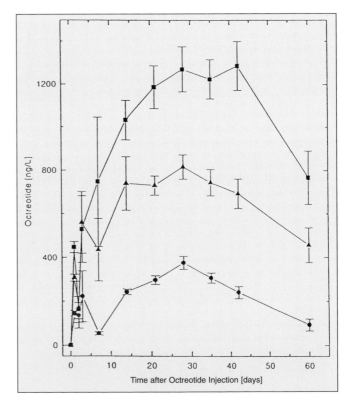

FIG. 67. Mean ± SEM octreotide concentrations vs. time profiles (on days 1, 7, 14, 21, 28, 35, 42, and 60) after administration of single doses of 10 mg (●; n = 16), 20 mg (▲; n = 39), or 30 mg (■; n = 37) octreotide to acromegalic patients. Each point is the mean of 12-h mean concentrations per patient. (From Lancranjan I, et al. Sandostatin LAR®: pharmacokinetics, pharmacodynamics, efficacy, and tolerability in acromegalic patients. *Metabolism* 1995;44: 18–26.)

demonstrating normalization of IGF-I levels. All patients experienced an improvement in clinical signs and symptoms (headache, sweating, fatigue, joint pain, carpal tunnel syndrome, and paresthesia). This formulation may be a very significant development in the medical treatment of acromegaly, allowing effective GH suppression while obviating the need for multiple daily injections. A slow-release version of lanreotide is also available (57).

Until the advent of long-acting somatostatin analogues, dopamine agonists (see below) represented the only effective medical therapy for acromegaly, reducing GH levels by more than 50% in 20–50% of patients (58,59). A number of comparative studies have now been performed with octreotide and bromocriptine in acromegaly. Direct comparisons have shown that octreotide provides better GH suppression than bromocriptine (60,61). However, when these drugs are given in combination, greater and more prolonged GH suppression has been noted than for each drug alone (62), although this has not been shown by others (63). This phenomenon is partially explained by the fact that octreotide co-administration increases the bioavailability of

bromocriptine by approximately 40% compared with bromocriptine's bioavailability when administered alone. The pharmacology of octreotide is unaffected during co-administration. Fløgstad et al. (62) noted that this may represent a possible mechanism for lowering GH and IGF-I levels more effectively while reducing the dose and frequency of administration of octreotide.

Effects of Octreotide on Signs and Symptoms

Large studies have shown that octreotide treatment improves signs and symptoms of acromegaly dramatically, in many cases before the improvement in biochemical parameters is significant. Headache, soft-tissue swelling, arthralgia, fatigue, and hyperhidrosis improve in up to 95% of acromegalic patients treated with octreotide, and improvement often occurs within the first few days of administration (Fig. 69). It is recognized that headache in acromegaly often responds extremely rapidly to octreotide, sometimes within hours of administration. This suggests that octreotide has a direct analgesic effect in these cases. Sleep apnea (64) has been shown to improve on octreotide therapy, although it is not known whether this is due to a decrease in upper airway resistance or whether central mechanisms are involved. Most significantly, however, cardiomyopathy has been shown to improve after octreotide treatment (65–67). Chanson et al. (68) reported that in a group of seven acromegalic patients, octreotide therapy led to an improvement in systemic arterial resistance, cardiac size, and exercise capacity within a few weeks. Lim and colleagues (69) reported a significant reduction in left ventricular mass within a week of starting octreotide in 10 acromegalic patients, an improvement that was sustained after 2 months of treatment. Interestingly, these authors noted that acromegalic patients without left ventricular hypertrophy experienced no change in ventricular size during octreotide treatment. Tokgözoglu et al. (70) reported a regression of left ventricular hypertrophy in six acromegalic patients treated with octreotide, in whom no secondary causes of left ventricular hypertrophy existed. Two patients had left ventricular hypertrophy at baseline, and the remaining four had wall thickness in the upper range of normal. Left ventricular mass decreased significantly in all patients, and treadmill exercise time and the maximal achievable heart rate increased significantly. Merola et al. (71) also reported improvements in functional cardiac diastolic filling parameters in acromegalic patients treated with octreotide for 6 months. The early-to-late peak left ventricular filling velocity was significantly correlated with a reduction in left ventricular mass. As outlined in an earlier chapter, mortality in acromegaly is determined to a large extent by cardiovascular disease. Improvement of underlying cardiac and respiratory pathology during octreotide treatment may therefore have a beneficial effect on life expectancy in acromegaly.

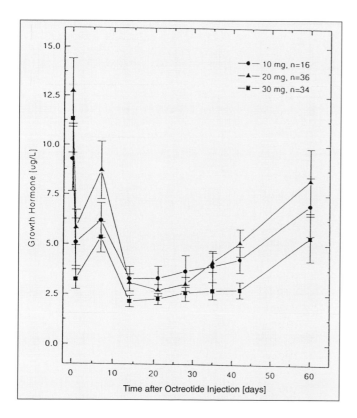

FIG. 68. Mean ± SEM GH concentrations vs. time profiles (on days 1, 7, 14, 21, 28, 35, 42, and 60) after administration of single doses of 10, 20, or 30 mg octreotide to acromegalic patients. Each point is the mean of 12-h mean concentrations per patient. (From Lancranjan I, et al. Sandostatin LAR®: pharmacokinetics, pharmacodynamics, efficacy, and tolerability in acromegalic patients. *Metabolism* 1995;44:18–26.)

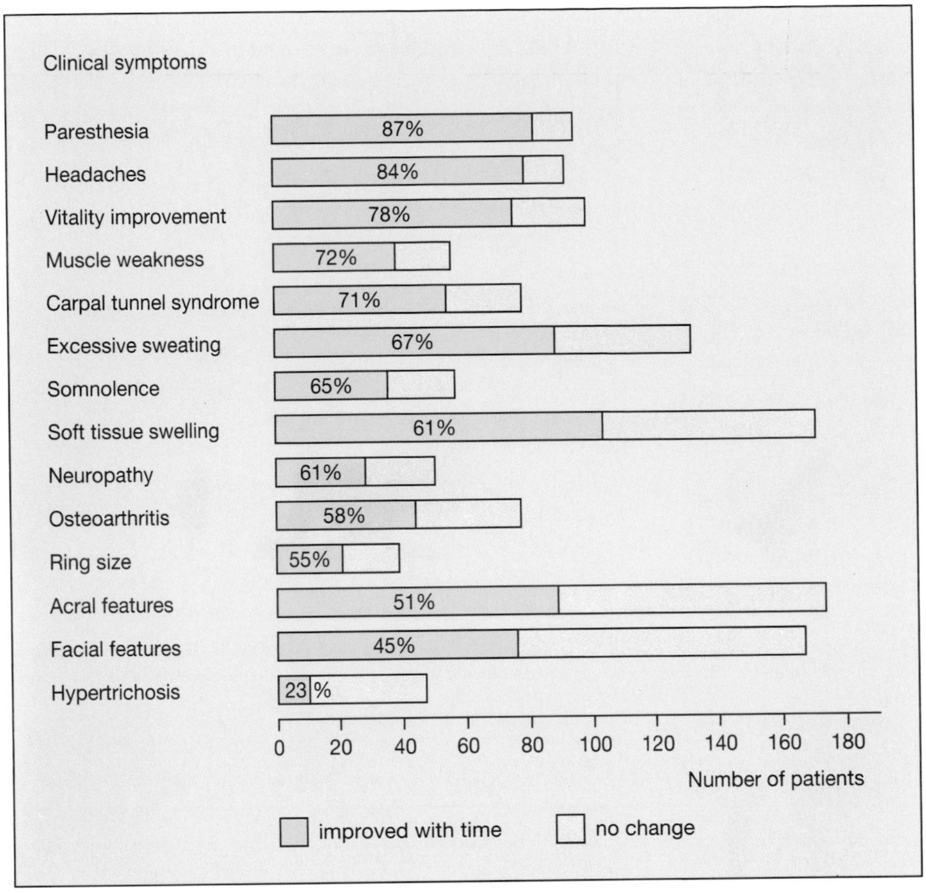

Clinical symptoms

Symptom	
Paresthesia	87%
Headaches	84%
Vitality improvement	78%
Muscle weakness	72%
Carpal tunnel syndrome	71%
Excessive sweating	67%
Somnolence	65%
Soft tissue swelling	61%
Neuropathy	61%
Osteoarthritis	58%
Ring size	55%
Acral features	51%
Facial features	45%
Hypertrichosis	23%

0 20 40 60 80 100 120 140 160 180
Number of patients

□ improved with time   □ no change

FIG. 69. Clinical improvement associated with octreotide therapy in 178 acromegalic patients. [From A.G. Harris et al., 1988 (45).]

TABLE 7. *Effect of octreotide on pituitary tumor size in patients with acromegaly*

Reference	Number of patients	Octreotide dose (μg/day)	Follow-up (weeks)	Number with pituitary shrinkage (%)
Barkan et al. (73)	10	300–1,000	3–30	10 (100)
Horikawa et al. (74)	8	600–800	3–38	6 (75)
Lund et al. (75)	10	≤1,500	75	10 (100)
Page et al. (76)	6	200–600	26	2 (33)
Sassolas et al. (43)	23	≤1,500	26	11 (48)
Stevenaert et al. (77)	32	300–1,500	12–156	19 (59.4)
	14	300	3–6	7 (50)
Ezzat et al. (44)	50	300	25	9 (19)
	54	750	25	20 (40)
Total	207			94 (45)

Adapted from C.A. Jaffe and A.L. Barkan, 1994 (80).

Pituitary Tumor Shrinkage

A very interesting phenomenon associated with octreotide therapy is pituitary tumor shrinkage, indicating that octreotide may be useful in the presurgical setting (Table 7). Approximately 40–50% of patients experience tumor size reduction, although the degree of shrinkage is highly variable (10–80%) (43,44,72–80) (Figs. 70–72). Morphologic changes may also occur with octreotide treatment, and it has been noted that some adenomas in octreotide-treated patients are softer and easier to resect. Shrinkage of a macroadenoma can lead to an improvement in vision as the tumor ceases to impinge on the optic chiasm. The morphologic changes that occur in pituitary tumors after octreotide therapy are variable (Table 8), but cytotoxic changes probably do not occur. Ezzat et al. (81) found no consistent morphologic changes in pituitary adenomas that could be attributable to octreotide treatment in tumors from

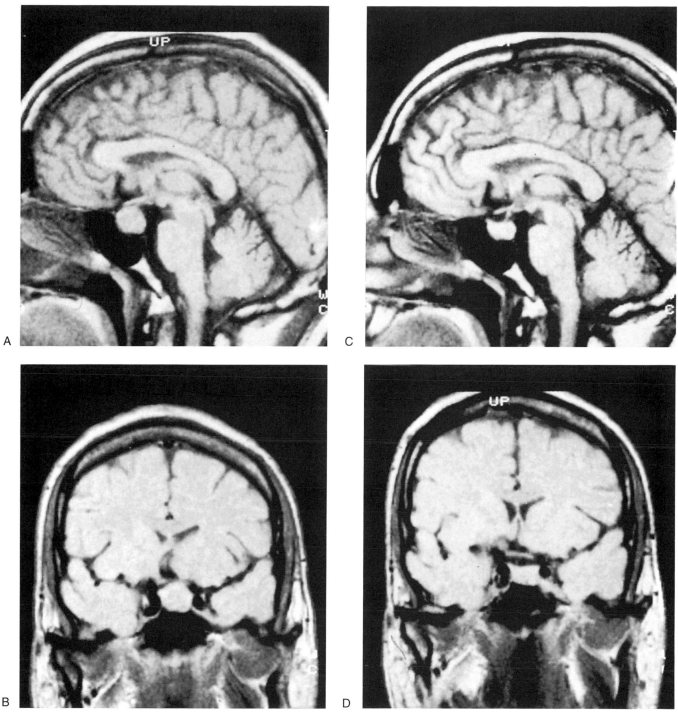

FIG. 70. MRI showing pituitary tumor shrinkage before and during octreotide therapy. (**A**) sagittal section before octreotide; (**B**) coronal section before octreotide; (**C**) sagittal section after octreotide; (**D**) coronal section after octreotide. (Courtesy of A. Stevenaert and A. Beckers.)

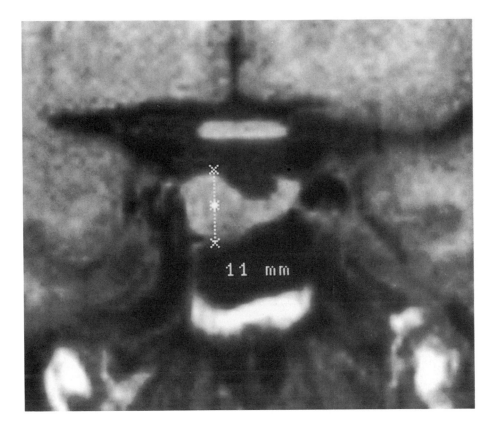

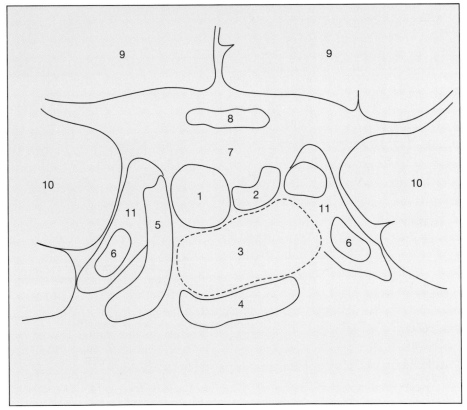

FIG. 71. MRI of a pituitary macro-adenoma before octreotide therapy. 1, Adenoma before octreotide therapy; 2, pituitary gland; 3, sphenoid sinus; 4, fat in the clinus; 5, carotid artery; 6, Meckel's cavity; 7, suprasellar cistern; 8, optic chiasm; 9, frontal lobe; 10, temporal lobe; 11, cavernous sinus. (Courtesy of A. Stevenaert and A. Beckers.)

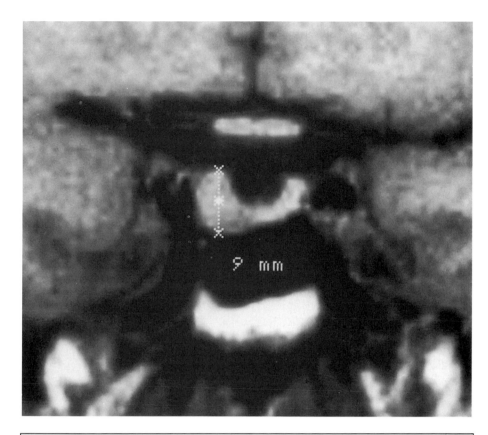

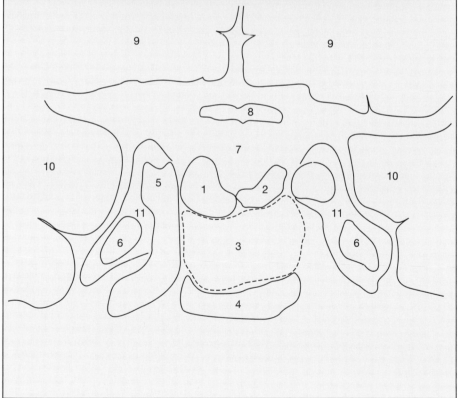

FIG. 72. MRI showing shrinkage of the pituitary macroadenoma during octreotide therapy. 1, Adenoma after octreotide therapy; 2, pituitary gland; 3, sphenoid sinus; 4, fat in the clinus; 5, carotid artery; 6, Meckel's cavity; 7, suprasellar cistern; 8, optic chiasm; 9, frontal lobe; 10, temporal lobe; 11, cavernous sinus. (Courtesy of A. Stevenaert and A. Beckers.)

TABLE 8. *Various morphological responses of pituitary adenoma tissue reported during octreotide therapy*

Increased cell diameter, cytoplasmic volume density of
  secretory granules (i.e., intracellular retention of GH)
Modest lysosomal accumulation, crinophagy
Cellular involution
Preservation of secretory apparatus with slight increase in
  GH immunoreactivity
Varying degrees of perivascular and interstitial fibrosis
No cellular change
No vascular change
No necrosis

86 acromegalic patients. One group (*n* = 43) of patients had undergone surgery after octreotide pretreatment, whereas another 43 patients received no pretreatment before surgery. Although perivascular and interstitial fibrosis was increased in the octreotide-treated tumors (72% vs. 42% of tumors), the authors noted no other striking morphologic changes, and tumor necrosis was not observed in any tumor treated with octreotide. In a recent study, Stevenaert and Beckers (82) reported that 59.7% of acromegalic patients experienced more than 25% tumor shrinkage after 3–6 weeks of treatment with octreotide. Remission rates in this series were significantly higher when the adenoma was enclosed rather than invasive (82). The main mechanism behind tumor shrinkage appears to be suppression of hormone release (83), probably coupled with increased intracellular breakdown of stored hormones, although a poor correlation between GH suppression and tumor shrinkage has been found (84).

The side effects of octreotide are usually transitory and mild in nature (Table 9), although an increased risk for gallstone formation has been extensively studied (52,85–87). About 25% of patients develop gallstones or biliary sludge during octreotide treatment, caused by an inhibitory effect of octreotide on gallbladder contraction and the promotion of biliary lithiasis. The condition is usually asymptomatic

TABLE 9. *Adverse events reported during octreotide therapy*

Local effects at injection site (last approximately 15 min)
  Pain
  Tingling/burning
  Redness
  Swelling
General adverse events (mainly gastrointestinal)
  Biliary sludge and cholelithiasis
  Anorexia
  Nausea and vomiting
  Abdominal cramp and/or bloating
  Loose stools
  Steatorrhea (no malabsorption)
  Hypoglycemia

and treatment may not be required. A consensus conference has stated that these gallstones should be managed similarly to gallstones in nonacromegalic patients, with ultrasound assessment and ursodeoxycholic acid treatment (88).

The place of octreotide (and other treatments) in the overall therapeutic protocol for acromegaly is illustrated in Fig. 73. Octreotide (100–200 μg s.c. every 6–8 h) is indicated in patients who are inadequately controlled by surgery and/or radiotherapy (or are waiting for the effects of radiotherapy to become apparent), and in patients who are unsuitable for surgical treatment. The effects of octreotide on tumor size and morphology outlined above raise the possibility of administering octreotide during the presurgical period. Finally, as Van der Lely et al. have noted (89), elderly patients have an excellent response to octreotide treatment, and it has been suggested that octreotide may be used as a primary treatment in older patients if they are unwilling or too infirm to undergo surgery.

Dopamine Agonists

The effect of dopamine agonist/ergot alkaloid agents such as bromocriptine on pituitary function has been studied for approximately 20 years (90). In normal subjects, L-dopa stimulates GH release. However, in the early 1970s it was noted that acromegalic patients had the opposite response to L-dopa, i.e., GH suppression (91). The precise site of action of dopamine agonists is still a matter of debate, but Jaffe and Barkan (92) have suggested that dopamine agonists have a bimodal effect, stimulating GH release at a central level and blocking GH release peripherally.

Bromocriptine can be administered orally because it is well absorbed from the gastrointestinal tract and is eliminated in bile via the liver. Jaffe and Barkan (92) have reviewed the results of 31 clinical trials using bromocriptine in the treatment of acromegaly (Fig. 74). They found that of 549 patients treated, approximately 20% had a GH level <5 μg/L, and only 10% had an IGF-I level in the normal range. Clinical response to bromocriptine treatment is reported by over 95% of patients, although improvements in physical features are often marginal. Headache, soft-tissue swelling, arthralgia, sleep apnea, and hyperhidrosis have all been reported to improve after bromocriptine therapy. Tumor shrinkage (often dramatic) occurs in many patients with prolactinomas who are treated with bromocriptine. However, the data concerning tumor shrinkage in acromegaly are not clear-cut. Approximately 30% of tumors were seen to shrink in Jaffe and Barkan's review of 10 studies. Interestingly, about 30% of tumors in acromegaly secrete GH and prolactin, and this may be the subset of adenomas in which bromocriptine causes tumor shrinkage. Side effects of bromocriptine treatment include nausea, postural hypotension, and constipation.

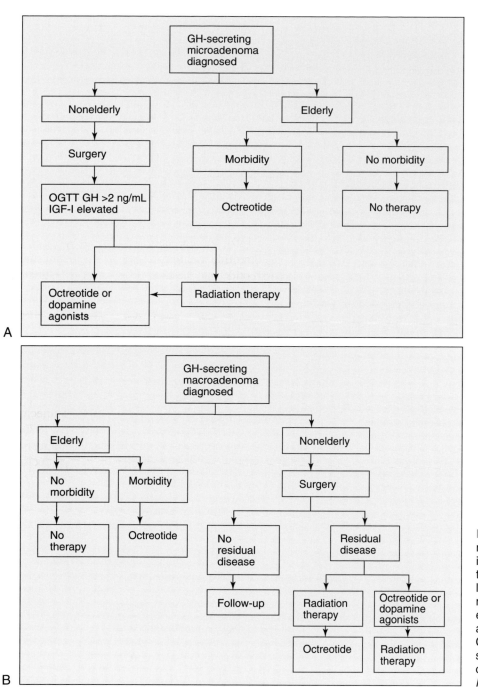

A

B

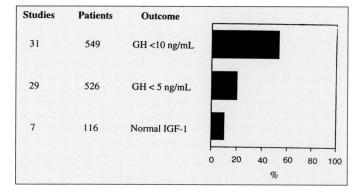

FIG. 73. Paradigms for the management of acromegaly caused by (A) pituitary microadenoma (<10 mm in diameter) and serum growth hormone (GH) levels <20 ng/ml; and by (B) macroadenoma (>10 mm in diameter) and GH levels >20 ng/ml. OGTT, oral glucose tolerance test. (From Acromegaly Therapy Consensus Development Panel. Consensus statement: benefits versus risks of medical therapy for acromegaly. *Am J Med* 1994;97:468.

FIG. 74. Percentage of acromegalic patients with GH levels below 5 or 10 ng/mL or normalized IGF-I levels after bromocriptine therapy. (From Melmed S, et al. Clinical review 75. Recent advances in pathogenesis, diagnosis, and management of acromegaly. *J Clin Endocrinol Metab* 1995;80:3395–402.)

A number of other dopamine agonists, such as terguride (93), cabergoline (94), pergolide (95), and CV 205-502 (96) have been developed, all of which have a longer half-life and fewer side effects than bromocriptine. None of these agents has demonstrated significant advantages over bromocriptine, other than requiring less frequent administration. Bromocriptine is also available in a depot formulation for patients who require chronic dopamine agonist therapy (97).

Given the moderate efficacy of dopamine agonists in the biochemical control of acromegaly, these agents are used as third-line treatments. Patients who have failed surgery and/or radiotherapy (or who are waiting for radiotherapy to become effective) and those who show no response to octreotide therapy can be considered for dopamine agonist treatment. It should be remembered that patients may experience greater disease control and more prolonged GH suppression with combined bromocriptine–octreotide administration than with either drug alone (see above), and this represents a valuable option in some acromegalic patients.

REFERENCES

1. Ho KY, Evans WS, Blizzard RM, et al. Effects of sex and age on the 24-hour profile of growth hormone secretion in man: importance of endogenous estradiol concentrations. *J Clin Endocrinol Metab* 1987;64:51–8.
2. Chapman IM, Hartman ML, Straue M, Johnson ML, Veldhuis JD, Thorner MO. Enhanced sensitivity growth hormone (GH) chemiluminescence assay reveals lower postglucose nadir GH concentrations in men than in women. *J Clin Endocrinol Metab* 1994;78:1312–9.
3. Cushing H. Partial hypophysectomy for acromegaly; with remarks on the function of the hypophysis. *Ann Surg* 1909;50:1002–17.
4. Parkinson D. A surgical approach to the cavernous portion of the carotid artery. Anatomical studies and case reports. *J Neurosurg* 1965;23:474–83.
5. Matsuno A, Sasaki T, Saito N, et al. Transcavernous surgery: an effective treatment for pituitary macroadenomas. *Eur J Endocrinol* 1995; 133:156–65.
6. Fahlbusch R, Honegger J, Buchfelder M. Surgical management of acromegaly. *Endocrinol Metab Clin North Am* 1992;21:669–92.
7. Hardy J, Somma M. Acromegaly: surgical treatment by transsphenoidal microsurgical removal of the pituitary adenoma. In: Tindall GT, Collins WF, eds. *Clinical management of pituitary disorders.* New York: Raven Press, 1979:209–17.
8. Laws ER, Randall RV, Abboud CF. Surgical treatment of acromegaly. Results in 140 patients. In: Givens JR, ed. *Hormone secreting pituitary tumours.* Chicago: Year Book Medical Publishers, 1982:225–8.
9. Teasdale GM, Hay ID, Beasttall GH, et al. Cryosurgery or microsurgery in the management of acromegaly. *JAMA* 1982;247:1289–91.
10. Grisoli F, Leclercq T, Jaquet P, Guibout M, Winteler JP, Hassoun J, Vincentelli F. Transsphenoidal surgery for acromegaly-long-term results in 100 patients. *Surg Neurol* 1985;23:513–19.
11. Landolt AM, Illig R, Zapf J. Surgical treatment of acromegaly. In: Lamberts SWJ, ed. *Sandostatin in the treatment of acromegaly.* Berlin: Springer-Verlag, 1988:23.
12. Ross DA, Wilson CB. Results of transsphenoidal microsurgery in for growth hormone-secreting pituitary adenomas in a series of 214 patients. *J Neurosurg* 1988;68:854–67.
13. Fahlbusch R, Honegger J, Buchfelder M. Surgical management of acromegaly. *Endocr Metab Clin North Am* 1992;21:669–91.
14. Tindall GT, Oyesiku NM, Watts NB, Clark RV, Christy JH, Adams PAC. Transsphenoidal adenomectomy for growth hormone-secreting pituitary adenomas in acromegaly: outcome analysis and determinants of failure. *J Neurosurg* 1993;78:205–15.
15. Davis DH, Laws ER, Ilstrup DM, et al. Results of surgical treatment for growth hormone-secreting pituitary adenomas. *J Neurosurg* 1993;79:70–5.
16. Zervas NT. Multicenter surgical results in acromegaly. In: Ludecke DK, Tolis G, eds. *Growth hormone, growth factors and acromegaly.* New York: Raven Press, 1987:253.
17. Ludecke DK. Recent developments in the treatment of acromegaly. *Neurosurg Rev* 1985;8:167–73.
18. Delalande O, Peillon F, Maestro JL, et al. Resultats a moyen et long terme de l'adenomectomie selective hypophysaire dand l'acromegalie: elements de prognostic. *Ann Endocrinol (Paris)* 1985;46:3213.
19. Fahlbusch J, Honegger J, Schott W, Buchfelder. Results of surgery in acromegaly. In: Wass JAH, ed. *Treating acromegaly.* Bristol, UK: Journal of Endocrinology Press, 1994:49–54.
20. Laws ER, Fode NC, Redmond MJ. Transsphenoidal surgery following unsuccessful prior therapy: an assessment of benefits and risks in 158 patients. *J Neurosurg* 1985;63:823.
21. Beclere A. The radio-therapeutic treatment of tumours of the hypophysis, gigantism and acromegaly. *Arch Roentgen Radiol* 1909;14:147.
22. Kliman B, Kjellberg RN, Swisher B, Butler W. *Acromegaly: a century of scientific and clinical progress.* New York: Plenum Press, 1987.
23. Speirs CJ, Reed PI, Morrison R, Aber V, Joplin GF. The effectiveness of external beam radiotherapy for acromegaly is not affected by previous ablative treatments. *Acta Endocrinol* 1990;122:559–65.
24. Feek CM, McLelland J, Seth J, et al. How effective is external pituitary irradiation for growth hormone-secreting pituitary tumors? *Clin Endocrinol* 1984;20:401–8.
25. Lamberg BA, Kivikangas V, Vartianen J, Raitta C, Pelkonen R. Conventional pituitary irradiation in acromegaly. Effect on growth hormone and TSH secretion. *Acta Endocrinol* 1976;82:267–81.
26. Eastman RC, Gorden P, Roth J. Conventional supervoltage irradiation is an effective treatment for acromegaly. *J Clin Endocrinol Metab* 1979;48:931–40.
27. Sheaves R. Pituitary irradiation for acromegaly. In: Wass JAH, ed. *Treating acromegaly.* Bristol, UK: Journal of Endocrinology Press, 1994:103–8.
28. Eastman RC, Gorden P, Glatstein E, Roth J. Radiation therapy of acromegaly. *Endocrinol Metab Clin North Am* 1992;21:693–712.
29. Jones A. Radiation oncogenesis in relation to the treatment of pituitary tumours. *Clin Endocrinol* 1991;35:379–97.
30. Brada M, Ford D, Ashley S, et al. Risk of second brain tumor after conservative surgery and radiotherapy for pituitary adenoma. *BMJ* 1992;304:1343–6.
31. Brada M, Rajan B. The toxicity of radiotherapy in the treatment of pituitary adenoma. In: Wass JAH, ed. *Treating acromegaly.* Bristol, UK: Journal of Endocrinology Press, 1994:127–32.
32. Jones A. Complications of radiotherapy for acromegaly. In: Wass JAH, ed. *Treating acromegaly.* Bristol, UK: Journal of Endocrinology Press, 1994:115–25.
33. Reubi JC, Landolt AM. The growth hormone responses to octreotide in acromegaly correlate with adenoma somatostatin receptor status. *J Clin Endocrinol Metab* 1989;68:844–50.
34. Guillemin R. Peptides in the brain: the new endocrinology of the neuron. *Science* 1978;202:390–402.
35. Sassolas G, Khalfallah Z, Chayvialle JA, et al. Effects of somatostatin analog BIM 23014 on the secretion of growth hormone, thyrotropin, and digestive peptides in normal men. *J Clin Endocrinol Metab* 1989;68:239–46.
36. Bauer W, Briner U, Doepfner W, et al. SMS 201-995: a very potent and selective octreotide analogue of somatostatin with prolonged action. *Life Sci* 1982;31:1133–40.
37. Bokser L, Schally AV. Delayed release formulation of the somatostatin analog RC-160 inhibits the growth hormone (GH) response to GH-releasing factor-(1–29) NH2 and decreases elevated prolactin levels in rats. *Endocrinology* 1988;123:1735–9.
38. Barkan AL, Kelch RP, Hopwood NJ, Beitins IZ. Treatment of acromegaly with the long-acting somatostatin analogue SMS 201-995. *J Clin Endocrinol Metab* 1988;66:16–23.
39. Lamberts SWJ, Oosterom R, Neufeld M, Del Pozo E. The somatostatin analog SMS 201-995 induces long acting inhibition of growth hormone hypersecretion in acromegalic patients. *J Clin Endocrinol Metab* 1985;60:1161–5.
40. Lamberts SWJ, Del Pozo E. Acute and long term effects of SMS 201-995 in acromegaly. *Scand J Gastroenterol* 1986;21:141–9.
41. Lamberts SWJ, Uitterlinden P, Verschoor L, van Dongen KJ, Del

Pozo E. Long term treatment of acromegaly with the somatostatin analogue SMS 201-995. *N Engl J Med* 1985;313:1576–80.

42. Lamberts SWJ, Uitterlinden P, Del Pozo E. Sandostatin (SMS 201-995) induces a continuous further decline in circulating growth hormone and somatomedin-C levels during therapy of acromegalic patients for over two years. *J Clin Endocrinol Metab* 1987;65:703–10.

43. Sassolas G, Harris AG, James-Dedier A, and the French SMS-201-995 Acromegaly Study Group. Long term effect of incremental doses of the somatostatin analog SMS 201-995 in 58 acromegalic patients. *J Clin Endocrinol Metab* 1990;71:391–7.

44. Ezzat S, Snyder PJ, Young WF, et al. Octreotide treatment of acromegaly: a randomized multicenter study. *Ann Intern Med* 1992;117:711–8.

45. Harris AG, Prestele H, Harold K, Boerlin V. Long term efficacy of Sandostatin (SMS 201-995, octreotide) in 178 acromegalic patients: results from the international multicenter acromegaly study group. In: Lamberts SWJ, ed. *Sandostatin in the treatment of acromegaly.* Berlin: Springer-Verlag, 1988:117–25.

46. Newman CB, Melmed S, Snyder PJ, et al. Safety and efficacy of long-term octreotide therapy of acromegaly: results of a multicenter trial in 103 patients—a clinical research center study. *J Clin Endocrinol Metab* 1995;80:2768–75.

47. Timsit J, Chanson PH, Larger E, et al. The effect of subcutaneous infusion versus subcutaneous injection of a somatostatin analogue (SMS 201-995) on the diurnal GH profile in acromegaly. *Acta Endocrinol* 1987;116:108–12.

48. Christensen SE, Weeke J, Orskov H, et al. Continuous subcutaneous pump infusion of a somatostatin analogue, SMS 201-995 versus subcutaneous injection schedule in acromegalic patients. *Clin Endocrinol* 1987;27:297–306.

49. James RA, White MC, Chatterjee S, Marciaj H, Kendall-Taylor P. A comparison of octreotide delivered by continuous subcutaneous infusion with intermittent injection in the treatment of acromegaly. *Eur J Clin Invest* 1992;22:554–61.

50. Roelfsema F, Frölien M, De Boer H, et al. Octreotide treatment of acromegaly: a comparison between pen-treated and pump-treated patients in a cross-over study. *Acta Endocrinol* 1991;125:43–8.

51. Tauber JP, Babin T, Ducasse MCR, Tauber MT, Harris AG, Bayard F. Long-term treatment of acromegaly by continuous subcutaneous infusion of the long-acting somatostatin analog Sandostatin (SMS 201-995, octreotide). In: Lamberts SWJ, ed. *Sandostatin in the treatment of acromegaly.* Berlin: Springer-Verlag, 1988:109–12.

52. Tauber JP, Poncet MF, Harris AG, et al. The impact of continuous subcutaneous infusion of octreotide on gallstone formation in acromegalic patients. *J Clin Endocrinol Metab* 1995;80:3262–6.

53. Weeke J, Christensen SE, Orskov H, et al. A randomized comparison of intranasal and injectable octreotide administration in patients with acromegaly. *J Clin Endocrinol Metab* 1992;75:163–9.

54. Fløgstad AK, Halse J, Haldorsen T, et al. Sandostatin LAR in acromegalic patients: a dose-ranging study. *J Clin Endocrinol Metab* 1995;80:3601–7.

55. Lancranjan I, Bruns C, Grass P, et al. Sandostatin LAR®: pharmacokinetics, pharmacodynamics, efficacy and tolerability in acromegalic patients. *Metab Clin Exp* 1995;44(suppl 1):18–26.

56. Kaal A, Frystyk J, Skjoerbaek C, et al. Effects of intramuscular microsphere-encapsulated octreotide on serum growth hormone, insulin-like growth factors (IGFs), free IGFs and IGF-binding proteins in acromegalic patients. *Metab Clin Exp* 1995;44(suppl 1):6–14.

57. Morange I, de-Boisvilliers F, Chanson P, et al. Slow release lanreotide treatment in acromegalic patients previously normalized by octreotide. *J Clin Endocrinol Metab* 1994;79:145–51.

58. Nortier JWR, Croughs RJM, Donker GH, Thijssen JHH, Schwarz F. Changes in plasma GH levels and clinical activity during bromocriptine therapy in acromegaly. The value of predictive tests. *Acta Endocrinol* 1984;106:175–83.

59. Chiodini PG, Cozzi R, Dallabonzana D, et al. Medical treatment of acromegaly with SMS 201-995, a somatostatin analog: a comparison with bromocriptine. *J Clin Endocrinol Metab* 1987;64:447–53.

60. Lamberts SWJ, Zwens M, Verschoor L, Del Pozo E. A comparison among the growth hormone lowering effects in acromegaly of the somatostatin analogue SMS 201-995, bromocriptine and the combination of both drugs. *J Clin Endocrinol Metab* 1986;63:16–9.

61. Wagenaar AH, Harris AG, van der Lely AJ, Lamberts SWJ. Dynamics of the acute effects of octreotide, bromocriptine and both drugs in combination on growth hormone secretion in acromegaly. *Acta Endocrinol* 1991;125:637–42.

62. Fløgstad AK, Halse J, Grass P, et al. A comparison of octreotide, bromocriptine, or a combination of both drugs in acromegaly. *J Clin Endocrinol Metab* 1991;79:461–5.

63. Fredstorp L, Lutz K, Werner S. Treatment with octreotide and bromocriptine in patients with acromegaly: an open pharmacodynamic interaction study. *Clin Endocrinol* 1994;41:103–8.

64. Grunstein RR, Ho KKY, Sullivan CE. Effect of octreotide, a somatostatin analog, on sleep apnea in patients with acromegaly. *Ann Intern Med* 1994;121:478–83.

65. Legrand V, Beckers A, Pham VT, Demoulin JC, Stevenaert A. Dramatic improvement of severe dilated cardiomyopathy in an acromegalic patient after treatment with octreotide and transsphenoidal surgery. *Eur Heart J* 1994;15:1286–9.

66. Thuesen L, Christensen SE, Weeke J, Orskov H, Henningsen P. The cardiovascular effects of octreotide treatment in acromegaly: an echocardiographic study. *Clin Endocrinol* 1989;30:619–25.

67. Pereira JL, Rodriguez-Puras MJ, Leal-Cerro A, et al. Acromegalic cardiopathy improves after treatment with increasing doses of octreotide. *J Endocrinol Invest* 1991;14:17–23.

68. Chanson P, Timsit J, Masquet C, et al. Cardiovascular effects of the somatostatin analogue octreotide in acromegaly. *Ann Intern Med* 1990;113:921–5.

69. Lim MJ, Barkan AL, Buda AJ. Rapid reduction of left ventricular hypertrophy in acromegaly after suppression of growth hormone hypersecretion. *Ann Intern Med* 1992;117:719–26.

70. Tokgözoglu SL, Erbas T, Aytemir K, Akalin S, Kes C, Oram E. Effects of octreotide on left ventricular mass in acromegaly. *Am J Cardiol* 1994;74:1072–4.

71. Merola B, Cittadini A, Colao A, et al. Chronic treatment with the somatostatin analog octreotide improves cardiac abnormalities in acromegaly. *J Clin Endocrinol Metab* 1993;77:790–3.

72. Barkan AL, Lloyd RV, Chandler WF, et al. Preoperative treatment of acromegaly with long-acting somatostatin analog SMS 201-995: shrinkage of invasive pituitary macroadenomas and improved surgical remission rate. *J Clin Endocrinol Metab* 1988;67:1040–8.

73. Horikawa R, Takano K, Hizuka N. Asakawa K, Sukegawa I, et al. Treatment of acromegaly with long-acting somatostatin analogue. SMS 20-1995. *Endocrinol Japonica* 1988;35:741–51.

74. Lund E, Jorgensen J, Christensen SE, Weeke J, Orskov H, Harris AG. Reduction in sella turcica volume: an effect of long-term treatment with the somatostatin analogue SMS 201-995 in acromegalic patients. *Neuroradiology* 1991;33:162–4.

75. Page MD, Millward ME, Taylor A, Preece M, Hourihan M, et al. Long-term treatment of acromegaly with a long-acting analog of somatostatin, octreotide. *Q J Med* 1991;274:189–201.

76. Stevenaert A, Harris AG, Kovacs K, Beckers A. Presurgical octreotide in acromegaly. *Metab Clin Exp* 1992;41(suppl 2):51–8.

77. Lucas-Morante T, Garcia-Uria J, Estrada J, et al. Treatment of invasive growth hormone secreting pituitary adenomas with long acting somatostatin analog SMS 201-995 before transsphenoidal surgery. *J Neurosurg* 1994;81:10–4.

78. Afshar F, Blackburn TPD, Huneidi AH. Transsphenoidal surgery versus octreotide treatment for acromegaly. In: Wass JAH, ed. *Treating acromegaly.* Bristol, UK: Journal of Endocrinology Press, 1994:55–7.

79. Ducasse MCR, Tauber JP, Tourre A, et al. Shrinking of a growth hormone-producing pituitary tumor by continuous subcutaneous infusion of the somatostatin analog, SMS 201-995. *J Clin Endocrinol Metab* 1987;65:1042–6.

80. Jaffe CA, Barkan AL. Acromegaly. Recognition and treatment. *Drugs* 1994;47:425–45.

81. Ezzat S, Horvath E, Harris AG, Kovacs K. Morphological effects of octreotide on growth hormone-producing pituitary adenomas. *J Clin Endocrinol Metab* 1994;79:113–8.

82. Stevenaert A, Beckers A. Presurgical octreotide treatment in acromegaly. *Acta Endocrinol* 1993;129(suppl 1):18–20.

83. Sautner D, Saeger W, Tallen G. Effects of octreotide on morphology of pituitary adenomas in acromegaly. *Pathol Res Pract* 1993;189:1044–51.

84. Plöckinger U, Reichel M, Fett U, Saeger W, Quabbe HJ. Preoperative octreotide treatment of growth hormone secreting and clinically nonfunctioning pituitary macroadenomas: effect on tumor volume and

lack of correlation with immunohistochemistry and somatostatin receptor scintigraphy. *J Clin Endocrinol Metab* 1994;79:1416–23.

85. Hussaini SH, Pereira SP, Murphy GM, et al. Composition of gall bladder stones associated with octreotide: response to oral ursodeoxycholic acid. *Gut* 1994;36:126–32.

86. Hussaini SH, Murphy GM, Kennedy C, Besser GM, Wass JAH, Dowling RH. The role of bile composition and physical chemistry in the pathogenesis of octreotide-associated gallbladder stones. *Gastroenterology* 1994;107:1503–13.

87. Redfern JS, Fortuner WJ. Octreotide-associated biliary tract dysfunction and gallstone formation: pathophysiology and management. *Am J Gastroenterol* 1995;90:1042–52.

88. Acromegaly Therapy Consensus Development Panel. Consensus statement: benefits versus risks of medical therapy for acromegaly. *Am J Med* 1994;97:468–73.

89. Van der Lely AJ, Harris AG, Lamberts SWJ. The sensitivity of growth hormone secretion to medical treatment in acromegalic patients: influence of age and sex. *Clin Endocrinol* 1992;37:181–5.

90. Chiodini PG, Liuzzi A, Botalla L, Oppizzi G, Muller EE, Silvestrini F. Stable reduction of plasma growth hormone (hGH) levels during chronic administration of 2-Br-alpha-ergocryptine (CB-154) in acromegalic patients. *J Clin Endocrinol Metab* 1975;40:705–8.

91. Liuzzi A, Chiodini PG, Botalla L, Cremascoli G, Silvestrini F. Inhibitory effect of L-dopa on GH release in acromegalic patients. *J Clin Endocrinol Metab* 1972;35:941–3.

92. Jaffe CA, Barkan AL. Treatment of acromegaly with dopamine agonists. *Endocrinol Metab Clin North Am* 1992;21:713–35.

93. Dallabonzana D, Liuzzi A, Oppizzi G, et al. Chronic treatment of pathological hyperprolactinemia and acromegaly with the new ergot-derivative terguride. *J Clin Endocrinol Metab* 1986;63:1002–7.

94. Ferrari C, Paracchi A, Romano C, et al. Long-lasting lowering of serum growth hormone and prolactin levels by single and repetitive cabergoline administration in dopamine-responsive acromegalic patients. *Clin Endocrinol* 1988;29:467–76.

95. Kleinberg DL, Boyd AG, Wardlow S, et al. Pergolide for the treatment of pituitary tumors secreting prolactin or growth hormone. *N Engl J Med* 1983;309:704–9.

96. Lombardi G, Colao A, Ferone D, et al. CV 205-502 treatment in therapy-resistant acromegalic patients. *Eur J Endocrinol* 1995;132:559–64.

97. Ciccarelli E, Miola C, Avataneo T, et al. Long-term treatment with a new repeatable injectable form of bromocriptine, parlodel LAR, in patients with tumorous hyperprolactinemia. *Fertil Steril* 1989;52:930–5.

CHAPTER 7

Acromegaly in Brief

Incidence: 3–4/million
Prevalence: 40–60/million
Mean age at onset: 32 years
Mean age at diagnosis: 39–42 years
Prognosis: Twofold increased mortality (due to cardiorespiratory disease and cancer)
Etiology and pathogenesis: Unrestrained GH secretion from a primary tumor of pituitary somatotropes (95%)
ectopic (<1%)
extrapituitary tumors (<1%)
excess GHRH secretion (<3%)

Diagnosis

Clinical Signs and Symptoms
Soft-tissue enlargement (macroglossia) and increased skin thickness
Coarsening of facial features
Skin tags
Oily skin
Hypertrichosis
Bony overgrowth [skull vault, sinuses, supraorbital ridges, lower jaw (prognathism)]
Increased interdental spaces
Malocclusion
Sleep apnea syndrome
Hypersomnolence
Carpal tunnel syndrome
Parasthesia
Kyphosis
Osteoarthritis
Arthralgia
Goiter
Cardiomyopathy/cardiomegaly
Hypertension
Fatigue

Effects of Pituitary Tumor Mass
Headache
Visual field defect
Cranial nerve involvement
Hypopituitarism

Biochemical Features
Serum GH fails to suppress to <2 μg/L following OGTT
Elevated IGF-I levels
Impaired glucose tolerance/diabetes mellitus
Elevated GHRH in ectopic GHRH-secreting tumor
Endocrine deficiencies

Imaging
Skull x-ray (enlarged sella, prognathism, enlarged sinuses)
CT/MRI (pituitary adenoma)

Management

Surgery
Transsphenoidal adenomectomy
Microadenomas (<10 mm diameter) 70–80% success
Invasive macroadenoma (>10 mm diameter) 30% success

Medical Therapy
Somatostatin analogues (octreotide 100–200 μg t.i.d.)
Clinical and biochemical response in up to 80% of patients
Tumor shrinkage in 40% of patients
Gallstones, sludge in 25% of patients
Dopamine agonists (e.g., bromocriptine up to 30 mg/day)
Control of GH secretion in up to 20% of patients
Gastrointestinal side effects, hypotension

Radiotherapy
Effective after 2–10 years
Requires concomitant medical therapy to control GH/IGF-I until GH falls
Side effects may be significant [hypopituitarism, second malignancy (?)]

Subject Index

Subject Index